SICK By DESIGN

HOW AMERICAN HEALTHCARE PRIORITIZES PROFIT OVER HEALTH

Studio 8 TwentyTwo, Sugar Land Texas

ISBN: 978-1-7362485-5-3

Library of Congress Control Number: 2026911678

To the patients the system failed, and the providers it broke trying to save them.

TABLE OF CONTENTS

DISCLAIMER

This book is intended for educational and informational purposes only. It does not constitute medical, legal, or financial advice.

The author is a licensed nurse practitioner, but this book does not create a patient-provider relationship with readers. Medical information presented is general in nature. Readers should consult their own healthcare providers for advice specific to their individual circumstances.

Patient stories in this book are composites based on the author's professional experience. Names, ages, genders, locations, diagnoses, timelines, and identifying details have been changed to protect patient privacy and ensure HIPAA compliance. Any resemblance to specific individuals is coincidental.

Statistical data, healthcare costs, and policy information were accurate at the time of publication but are subject to change. Readers should verify current information through official sources before making healthcare or financial decisions.

This book contains the author's opinions and analysis regarding the American healthcare system, insurance companies, pharmaceutical companies, government policies, and public figures. These views are based on the author's professional experience, research, and publicly available information. They do not represent the views of any employer, professional organization, or licensing board. Criticism of corporations, policies, and public figures reflects the author's constitutionally protected right to free speech on matters of public concern.

Neither the author nor the publisher makes any guarantees regarding the completeness or accuracy of the information in this book, nor assumes liability for actions readers take based on this information. Readers are responsible for their own healthcare, financial, and legal decisions and should consult qualified professionals as needed.

Author's Note on The Currency of Information

I completed this manuscript in January 2026. Every statistic, policy detail, and legislative reference was accurate at that time, using the most recent data available from government sources, peer-reviewed research, and reputable health policy organizations. I updated the manuscript in March 2026 to reflect the most current healthcare spending data across nations.

However, American healthcare is a rapidly moving target. Laws change. Policies shift. Administrations come and go, each with different priorities and approaches to healthcare regulation—and different levels of transparency about the data they release. The Affordable Care Act has been under constant threat since its passage. Medicaid expansion remains a political battleground. Insurance regulations, subsidy programs, and coverage requirements can change with a single vote in Congress or a stroke of an executive pen.

The fundamental arguments in this book—about how the system was designed, who it serves, and why it functions as it does—remain true regardless of which party controls what branch of government. But specific details, particularly around current policies and spending figures, may have changed between when I finished writing and when you're reading this.

If you need current, reliable information for making healthcare decisions or understanding policy changes, I recommend checking:

- **Peer-reviewed medical and health policy journals** (JAMA, The Lancet, Health Affairs, New England Journal of Medicine)

- **Single-payer advocacy organizations** that track healthcare data independently (Physicians for a National Health Program, Healthcare-NOW!)

- **Independent health policy research organizations** (Kaiser Family Foundation, Commonwealth Fund, Peterson-KFF Health System Tracker)

- **Academic medical centers and schools of public health** that publish healthcare research and policy analysis

For the most reliable and unbiased information, prioritize peer-reviewed research and independent health policy organizations over government press releases.

What won't change: the fact that American healthcare remains uniquely expensive, uniquely fragmented, and uniquely capable of bankrupting people for the crime of getting sick. That's not a temporary policy position. That's by design.

—Nachole Johnson

March 2026

INTRODUCTION

I was sitting in my car on my lunch break, scrolling through YouTube, when I saw the headline: *"United Healthcare CEO Brian Thompson Shot and Killed Outside Manhattan Hotel."*

When it came out that it wasn't just a random shooting, but a targeted attack, I knew exactly why.

Not the specific grievances of the shooter. Not the details that would emerge later—the bullet casings engraved with "deny," "defend," "depose." Not the manifesto or the backstory. I didn't know any of that yet.

But I knew *why*.

I'm a nurse practitioner. I've worked in hospitals, insurance companies, urgent care clinics, and private practices. I've seen the system from every angle. At that moment, sitting in my car with fifteen minutes left before I had to go back inside, I felt something I'm ashamed to admit: I had no empathy for Brian Thompson.

I'm a Christian woman. I believe in the sanctity of human life. I grieve violence. Yet when I heard that a healthcare CEO had been killed, my first thought wasn't sorrow—it was understanding.

When I walked back into the clinic that afternoon, my colleagues were shocked. "Who would do something like this?" they kept asking. "What kind of person murders someone in cold blood?"

I stayed silent. Because my answer—*millions of Americans who've been denied, delayed, and bankrupted by the system he profited from*—wasn't something I could say out loud. Not there. Not as a practicing provider who still had to work within this system to pay my own bills.

But here's what terrified me most about that moment: I wasn't alone in my reaction.

Within hours, the internet exploded—not with mourning, but with memes. With jokes. With barely concealed satisfaction. The wanted poster for the shooter generated more sympathy than outrage. People shared their own denial stories, their bankruptcy stories, their "my loved one died waiting for prior authorization" stories. The collective response wasn't "how horrible"—it was *"I understand."*

A CEO was dead, and America's response was a dark, bitter: Finally.

That should horrify us. Not because violence is ever the answer—it isn't. It should horrify us because it reveals just how deep the rot goes. When millions of people see a healthcare executive gunned down and their first reaction is understanding rather than shock, we're not looking at a public relations problem. We're looking at a moral reckoning.

The assassination of an insurance CEO didn't break the American healthcare system. It revealed what's been true all along: the system was already broken. Or more accurately, it was never broken at all.

It's working exactly as designed.

Who I Am & Why I'm Writing

My name is Nachole Johnson.

I'm a nurse practitioner with over twenty years of experience in the American healthcare system. I've worked in hospitals, insurance companies, urgent care clinics, and private practices. I've seen this system from every angle.

I can't stay silent anymore.

I've worked in hospitals where we admitted patients who couldn't afford their medications. I've worked in urgent care clinics where patients came in desperately sick because they didn't have a primary care provider—or insurance to see one. I've worked in private practices where patients making six figures still asked me, nervously, how much the visit would cost.

I've even worked for a major insurance company doing home visits.

That's where I saw how the machine really works. Not from the bedside, where you see the human cost, but from inside the system that creates that cost. Billing teams constantly asking if there were additional diagnoses to document. Pressure to maximize reimbursement codes. The incentive structure rewarded finding problems, not preventing them—because every billable condition, every complication documented, every code captured meant higher reimbursement.

It wasn't fraud. It was the revenue model. It was how you kept the doors open.

It felt uncomfortable, but it was legal. It was normal.

I told myself I was helping people.

I was.

But I was also part of a predatory system that extracts maximum profit from human suffering.

That's what I mean when I say I feel like I'm on the wrong side. Not because I'm a bad person—I don't think most people working in healthcare are bad people. Because the system itself is designed to profit from sickness, not health. And everyone who works within it—insurers, hospital administrators, pharmaceutical executives, and yes, even providers like me—become complicit in that design.

I grew up using free clinics. My mother took my brother and I when we were sick because we couldn't afford anything else. I got my braces at a dental school because, once again, we couldn't afford them from an established orthodontist. When I got my first nursing job as an LPN (licensed practical nurse) at twenty and finally had health insurance, I was afraid to use it. I didn't understand deductibles or copays or out-of-pocket maximums—I just knew that having insurance didn't mean healthcare was free, and I was terrified of ending up with a bill I couldn't pay.

Years later, when I needed major surgery, I had insurance through my employer. Their best plan had a $6,000 deductible. Six. Thousand. Dollars. The surgery itself was billed at over $70,000, so I know I was lucky—insurance "saved" me $64,000. But I was a healthcare provider with a good job and decent insurance, and I still had to come up with $6,000 to have a life-saving surgery. Coming up with six thousand dollars is a lot for the average American.

If that's the system working, we need a new system.

I'm writing this book because I'm tired of watching people suffer. I'm tired of the apologetic conversations where patients ask if they really need that test, that medication, that follow-up appointment—not because they don't want to get better, but because they're trying to calculate whether they can afford it. I'm tired of watching people making $100,000 a year worry about the same thing as people making $30,000 a year: *What happens if I get sick?*

Most of all, I'm tired of pretending this is normal. That it's acceptable. That healthcare is a privilege to be earned rather than a right to be guaranteed.

I can't fix this system alone. I can name it, though. I can explain how it works, why it works this way, and who it's designed to serve. I can tell the truth about what I've seen from the inside.

I know this is uncomfortable. But here's what needs to be said:

The American healthcare system is not broken. It is not failing. It is not in need of minor repairs or incremental improvements.

It is working exactly as designed.

When I say "designed," I don't mean there was a secret meeting where evil executives plotted to make people suffer. I mean that every single feature of our healthcare system—every incentive, every structural choice, every policy decision—was built to serve specific interests. The problem is that those interests were never about keeping Americans healthy.

The healthcare system was designed on a foundation of racial exclusion. When the federal government funded hospital construction in 1946, it explicitly allowed those hospitals to be segregated. When employer-based insurance became the norm, it deliberately excluded the jobs Black Americans were most likely to hold—agricultural work, and domestic service. The resistance to "universal" healthcare wasn't about economics or freedom—it was about avoiding integration and redistribution.

The system was designed to maximize profit, not health. Insurance companies make money by collecting premiums and denying claims. Pharmaceutical companies make money by keeping drugs expensive and patents perpetual. Hospitals make money by treating complications, not preventing them. The entire financial model depends on you getting sick and staying sick, not on keeping you well.

The system was designed to be reactive, not preventive. There's no money in stopping you from getting diabetes. On the other hand, there's enormous money in managing your diabetes for thirty years—insulin, test strips, doctor visits, eventual complications, dialysis, amputations. Prevention pays once. Disease management pays forever.

The system was designed to fragment, not universalize. Employer-based insurance keeps you tied to your job, fearful of leaving, unable to start a business or take a risk. Medicaid eligibility varies by state, often along racial lines. Medicare covers seniors but not their adult children. Every gap, every complexity, every bureaucratic barrier serves someone's interest—just not yours.

This isn't a conspiracy theory. This is documented history and observable reality. Once you see the design, you can't unsee it.

The question isn't "How do we fix the broken healthcare system?" The question is: "Are we willing to dismantle a system that's working exactly as intended—for insurance companies, pharmaceutical executives, hospital administrators, and politicians who take their money?"

Because that's what it will take. Not reform, not tweaks, not incremental improvements.

We need to tear it down and build something designed for a different purpose: keeping people healthy, not extracting profit from their suffering.

That's what this book is about. Not how the system failed, but how it succeeded—and why that success looks like cruelty to everyone who isn't profiting from it.

What Happened to Brian Thompson

December 4, 2024, was a Wednesday morning. Brian Thompson, CEO of UnitedHealthcare, was walking to an investor conference in Manhattan when a masked gunman shot him multiple times and fled on an electric bike.

The shooter left behind bullet casings engraved with three words: "Deny. Defend. Depose."

Within hours, those three words became a rallying cry.

Not because Americans celebrated violence—though the media tried desperately to frame it that way. But it was because those three words named something that millions of people had experienced but never heard acknowledged by anyone in power: the systematic cruelty of an industry that profits by saying "no."

Deny the claim. Defend the denial. Depose anyone who challenges it in court.

That's the playbook. And everyone knew it.

I watched the response unfold in real time, and what struck me wasn't the memes or the jokes—though there were plenty. What struck me was the sheer volume of personal stories that poured out. Story after story of people who had been denied coverage for life-saving treatments. Of people who had died waiting for prior authorization. Of people who had done everything right—had insurance, paid their premiums, followed the rules—and still ended up bankrupted or dead.

These weren't fringe conspiracy theorists. These were ordinary Americans, sharing their experiences with a system that had failed them so profoundly that when a CEO was murdered, their first response was: *I understand why.*

The media called it disturbing. Politicians called it unacceptable. Healthcare executives clutched their pearls and hired private security.

But nobody asked the obvious question: *Why are millions of Americans not surprised that someone killed a healthcare CEO?*

The answer is simple: because the system kills people every single day, and nobody with power seems to care.

UnitedHealthcare—Thompson's company—has the highest claim

denial rate in the industry. Let that sink in for a moment. People pay $500, $800, $1,200 per month or more in premiums—money that comes out of every single paycheck, whether they use healthcare that month or not. For a family, that's often $15,000 to $20,000 per year just for the privilege of having insurance.

Then, when they actually get sick and need the coverage they've been paying for, UnitedHealthcare denies their claims at higher rates than any other major insurer.

They use an AI algorithm to auto-deny claims, then make patients fight through appeals processes designed to exhaust them into giving up. They delay authorizations for treatments their own doctors recommend. They terminate coverage mid-treatment. They do everything in their power to avoid paying for the care they contractually promised to cover—care that patients have already paid thousands of dollars to access.

And this is legal. All of it.

Thompson wasn't some rogue executive operating outside the law. He was doing exactly what the system rewards: maximizing shareholder value by minimizing payouts. Under his leadership, UnitedHealthcare's profits soared. Wall Street loved him. Investors praised him. He was successful by every metric that matters in American healthcare.

All measures except one: keeping people alive and healthy.

The day Thompson died, UnitedHealthcare's stock barely moved. The company issued a perfunctory statement about tragedy and loss, then got back to business. Because in American healthcare, no individual—not even a CEO—is more important than the profit model.

That's what people understood when they saw the news. Not that violence was justified—but that his death was a symptom of the very same system that kills their family members, their friends, and their neighbors. A system where human life is a line item on a balance sheet, to be minimized for maximum profit.

The memes weren't celebrating murder. They were expressing something darker and more desperate: the recognition that nothing else had worked. Not protests, not petitions, not elections. Not even exposés, investigations, or lawsuits. The system kept grinding forward, denying claims, bankrupting families, letting people die—all while executives got richer and politicians took their donations and nothing fundamentally changed.

When the only response to systematic cruelty is systematic indifference, people stop believing in the possibility of change through official channels.

That's not a justification for violence. It's a diagnosis of social collapse.

And the response from people in power? They didn't ask why Americans were so angry. They didn't question whether a system that generates this much rage might need fundamental reform. They hired more security guards and went back to business as usual.

I want to be clear: I don't condone what happened to Brian Thompson. I don't believe violence is the answer. I believe in working within systems to change them, in advocacy and organizing and policy reform.

That said, I also understand why millions of Americans saw that news and thought: *Finally, someone who profits from this system faced a consequence*.

That's the real story of December 4, 2024. Not that a CEO was killed, but that a nation collectively shrugged and said: *What did you expect?*

This book exists because of that moment. Because the mask slipped, and we all saw what we'd been pretending not to see: that the American healthcare system isn't just failing—it's predatory. And people are so desperate, so exhausted, so financially and emotionally devastated by it that when violence erupts, they understand it.

We can't go back to pretending everything is fine. We can't keep accepting "this is just how it works" as an answer. We can't keep letting people die for profit and calling it healthcare.

The insurance CEO assassination didn't start the conversation about American healthcare, but it made the conversation impossible to ignore.

That's why I'm writing this book now.

What This Book Will Show You

This book is divided into four parts, and each one builds on the last.

Part I: The Foundation takes you back to where this all started. Not last year or last decade, but to the deliberate policy choices that built American healthcare on a foundation of racial exclusion. You'll learn about the Hill-Burton Act of 1946, which used federal dollars to fund segregated hospitals. You'll understand how employer-based insurance was designed to exclude Black workers. You'll see why "universal healthcare" became politically toxic—because universal meant integration, and integration meant redistribution. The racism isn't incidental to American healthcare. It's foundational.

Part II: The Current Crisis shows you how that foundation evolved into the predatory machine we have today. You'll understand why insurance companies profit more from denying your claims than paying them—even after you've paid thousands in premiums. You'll see why the system rewards reactive treatment over prevention, chronic disease management over cures, and complexity over simplicity. You'll learn why medical bankruptcy is the leading cause of bankruptcy in America, why two-thirds of those families had insurance when they got sick, and why entrepreneurs and small business owners are trapped in jobs they hate because leaving means losing healthcare.

Part III: The Resistance examines the breaking points; the CEO assassination; the ongoing attacks on the Affordable Care Act; the provider burnout epidemic that's driving healthcare workers out of the profession in record numbers—not because the work is hard, but because the moral injury of participating in a predatory system becomes unbearable. You'll understand why the public response to December 4th wasn't shock—it was recognition.

Part IV: What We Deserve lays out what's possible. Not utopian fantasy, but observable reality in every other developed nation. You'll see how preventative care actually works, what it costs, and what it returns. You'll understand the different models of universal healthcare and why the "but how will we pay for it?" question is backwards—we're already paying more than anyone else in the world for worse outcomes. The question isn't whether we can afford universal healthcare—it's whether we can afford to keep this system.

By the end of this book, you'll have the necessary insight to understand three things:

First, the American healthcare system isn't broken—it's working exactly as intended, and perfectly for the people it was built to serve.

Second, you're not crazy for being angry. The rage you feel when you get a denial letter, when you're afraid to call an ambulance, when you stay in a job you hate for the insurance—that's a rational response to irrational cruelty.

Third, it doesn't have to be this way. Every other developed nation has figured this out. We can too.

First, though, we have to be willing to see the system for what it is.

A Note on Stories

Throughout this book, you'll read stories from my years working in healthcare. Some are drawn from my personal experience—my own medical bills, my time working inside an insurance company, patterns I witnessed as a practicing nurse practitioner. Others are composite scenarios constructed to illustrate systemic problems I encountered repeatedly.

When you read about Marcus, the graphic designer trapped in his job by a preexisting condition, or Maria, the entrepreneur who lost her coverage—these individuals may not exist as described. The situations they face, however, are real. I've watched these scenarios play out hundreds of times with different names, different diagnoses, different details. The specifics change. The harm is consistent.

Some stories come from aggregated data—like the real premium costs shared by real Americans in online discussions, or the bankruptcy statistics documented in peer-reviewed research. These aren't my patients. They're examples of systemic dysfunction that affects millions.

Where I do draw from clinical experience, I've removed any identifying details that could connect a story to a real person. This isn't to obscure the truth—it's to protect it. HIPAA laws exist for good reason, and I take patient privacy seriously. More than that, I take my responsibility as a healthcare provider seriously, even when I'm writing a book.

The core of every story—the systemic failure, the financial devastation, the moral injury, the bureaucratic cruelty—is real. These failures are documented throughout this book with citations from peer-reviewed research, government data, and policy analysis. The emotional truth is intact because the systemic harm is constant.

I'm telling you this upfront because I want you to trust what you're reading. These aren't exaggerated anecdotes designed to manipulate your emotions. They're not cherry-picked worst-case scenarios. They're representative examples of what happens every single day in American healthcare, to millions of people, in ways that are so normalized we've stopped registering them as cruelty.

The question isn't whether any specific Marcus or Maria existed exactly as described. The question is whether the American healthcare system routinely traps people in jobs they want to leave, bankrupts families despite insurance, denies necessary care to maximize profit, and burns out providers who can't reconcile participation in a predatory system with their commitment to healing.

The answer—backed by research, documented by data, and confirmed by my years of clinical experience—is yes.

The data in this book is meticulously sourced. Every statistic, every policy detail, every historical fact is cited and verifiable. You can check my work. You *should* check my work.

However, data alone doesn't capture what it feels like to watch someone ration insulin because they can't afford their prescription. Numbers don't convey the expression on a patient's face when you tell them their insurance denied coverage for the treatment they need. Statistics can't explain what it does to a healthcare provider's soul to be part of a system that forces those conversations.

That's why the stories matter. Not as proof—but as a witness.

I've seen what this system does to people. I've been complicit in it, and I can't stay silent about it anymore.

The stories are anonymized. The anger is not.

Who This Book Is For

This book is for anyone who has ever been afraid to call an ambulance because of the cost.

It's for anyone who has stayed in a job they hate because leaving means losing health insurance.

It's for anyone who has gotten a medical bill and felt their stomach drop, even though they have insurance and thought they were covered.

It's for the entrepreneurs who can't start their businesses because they can't risk losing coverage. For the parents who ration their own medications so their kids can have what they need. For the people making $100,000+ a year who are still one serious illness away from bankruptcy.

It's for healthcare workers who are exhausted—not from the work itself, but from the moral injury of participating in a system that prioritizes profit over patients. For the nurses who watch people suffer needlessly. For the doctors who spend more time fighting insurance companies than treating patients. For everyone who went into healthcare to help people and discovered they're working for a machine designed to extract maximum revenue from human suffering.

It's for anyone who saw the news about the assassination and understood, immediately, why it happened—even if you couldn't say that out loud.

It's for people who are tired of being told the system is too complicated to understand, too expensive to fix, too entrenched to change. For people who know something is deeply wrong but can't quite articulate what or why.

This book is for you if you've ever thought: *This can't be normal. This can't be how it's supposed to work. Other countries don't do it this way—why do we?*

You're right. It's not normal. It's not supposed to work this way. Other countries don't do it this way because they designed their systems differently, with different goals and different values.

We can too.

But first, I need you to understand how we got here, why the system works the way it does, and who benefits from keeping it exactly as broken as it appears.

That's what this book will show you.

I'm going to make you angry.

That's not a warning—it's a promise. If you finish this book and you're not furious, I haven't done my job.

But here's the thing about anger: it's not a problem to be managed. It's information to be trusted. Your rage at a system that bankrupts families, denies life-saving care, and profits from suffering isn't irrational—it's the only sane response to institutionalized cruelty.

For too long, we've been told that anger about healthcare is unproductive. That we need to be reasonable, pragmatic, willing to compromise. That change takes time and we should be grateful for incremental progress.

I'm done with that. You should be too.

The people profiting from this system aren't being reasonable. Insurance companies aren't compromising when they deny your claims. Pharmaceutical executives aren't being pragmatic when they charge $300 for insulin that costs $10 to produce. Politicians aren't grateful for your patience while they take campaign donations from the industry that's killing you.

So yes, this book will make you angry. It will show you exactly how the system was designed, who designed it, and why they designed it to work against you. It will name the mechanisms of exploitation and the people who profit from them.

But I won't leave you there.

Part IV of this book is about what we deserve and how we get it. Not fantasy, but reality—the reality that exists in every other developed nation, where people don't die because they can't afford insulin, where medical bankruptcy doesn't exist, where healthcare is treated as a human right instead of a profit center.

This book will validate your anger, explain where it comes from, and show you that the fury you feel isn't just justified—it's necessary. Because anger is what fuels change, and this system desperately needs to change.

So let's talk about how American healthcare was built on a foundation of racism, perfected by greed, and maintained through deliberate cruelty.

Let's talk about why it works exactly as designed.

Then, we'll talk about what it will take to tear it down and build something better.

PART 1

THE FOUNDATION

CHAPTER 1

The Foundation Built on Exclusion

These opening scenarios are hypothetical, constructed to illustrate a common reality.

Sarah worked as a marketing manager for a tech startup in Austin. Good job, good salary, good health insurance through her employer. When she got pregnant, her insurance covered her prenatal care, her delivery, everything. Six months after her daughter was born, the startup folded. Sarah lost her job—and her health insurance—overnight.

She immediately applied for coverage through the Affordable Care Act marketplace. Her new premium? $850 a month for a plan with a $7,000 deductible. On unemployment benefits, she couldn't afford it. She made too much for Medicaid in Texas, which hadn't expanded the program. So she went without insurance, skipped her postpartum follow-up appointments, and prayed nothing went wrong with her or her baby until she found another job with benefits.

Michael worked as a restaurant manager in Wisconsin— a stable job; been there eight years. The company health plan covered him and his wife. When a larger chain acquired his company, his insurance changed. The new plan didn't cover his wife's rheumatologist—the doctor she'd been seeing for five years to manage her lupus. They could pay out-of-network rates ($400 per visit instead of $40) or switch doctors and start over with someone new who might not be as familiar with her case.

They switched doctors. The new rheumatologist changed her medication protocol. Three months later, she ended up hospitalized with a lupus flare that landed them with $15,000 in medical bills—bills their old insurance would have covered differently, bills they're still paying off two years later.

Lisa lives in Virginia, right on the border with Tennessee. She works as a home health aide, making $32,000 a year. In Virginia, that's just above the Medicaid income threshold—she makes too much to qualify. If she lived fifteen miles south in Tennessee, she'd be eligible for Medicaid coverage. Instead, she goes without insurance, treats her diabetes with Walmart insulin she can barely afford, and hasn't seen a doctor in three years.

Three different people. Three different situations. One common thread: their access to healthcare depends entirely on their employment status, their employer's decisions, and which state they happen to live in.

This is the American healthcare system. And it is utterly insane.

No other developed nation structures healthcare this way. In Canada, your coverage doesn't disappear when you lose your job. In Germany, your doctor doesn't change when your employer switches insurance companies. In the United Kingdom, healthcare access doesn't depend on which side of an arbitrary state line you live on.

The United States spends more on healthcare than any other nation in the world—and it's not even close.

In 2024, the U.S. spent $14,775 per person on healthcare—17.2% of our entire economy. Compare that to other wealthy nations: peer countries including Australia, Austria, Belgium, Canada, France, Germany, Japan, Netherlands, Sweden, Switzerland, and the United Kingdom averaged $7,860 per capita—about half of what the U.S. spends. We spend nearly double what comparable nations spend, and projections show U.S. healthcare consuming 20.3% of GDP by 2033.

No other developed nation dedicates more than 12% of their GDP to healthcare. Peer countries average 11.2% of GDP. The U.S. spends 17.2%—more than 50% higher than peer nations.

You might think that massive spending buys us the best healthcare in the world. World-class outcomes. Longer lives. Healthier populations.

It doesn't.

U.S. life expectancy is 76.4 years. By comparison, Canada's is 82.7 years. Japan's is 84.8 years. Spain's is 83.2 years. By 2021, fifty-six countries on six continents had surpassed U.S. life expectancy—not just other wealthy nations, but countries like Costa Rica, Chile, and Slovenia. Americans live shorter lives than people in countries spending half of what we do.

And that gap is widening. Between 2010 and 2020, the life expectancy gap between the U.S. and peer countries grew from

1.88 years to 4.69 years. We're not falling behind slowly—we're dropping off a cliff.

Our infant mortality rate is worse than nearly every developed nation. For every 1,000 babies born in the United States, 5.6 die before their first birthday. In Germany, that number is 3.1. In Japan, it's 1.8. In Finland—which has the lowest rate—it's 1.7. American babies are 1.78 times more likely to die in their first year than babies in other OECD (The Organisation for Economic Co-operation and Development) countries.

Here's what should enrage you: even the most privileged White Americans in the top 1% wealthiest counties have an infant mortality rate of 3.54 per 1,000—still higher than the national average in all twelve comparison countries except Canada. Even our richest, most advantaged citizens can't buy their way to outcomes that are normal everywhere else.

Maternal mortality tells an even grimmer story. Between 2018 and 2022, U.S. maternal mortality increased from 25.3 to 32.6 deaths per 100,000 live births—a 27.7% increase in just four years. That makes the U.S. maternal death rate two to four times higher than other high-income countries. In Canada, it's 11.2 per 100,000. In Germany, it's 4. In Japan, it's 4. American mothers are seven to eight times more likely to die from pregnancy-related complications than mothers in other wealthy countries.

For Black mothers in America, the rate is 69.9 per 100,000—two to three times higher than for White women, and worse than many developing nations. Two-thirds of these deaths are preventable.

These aren't marginal differences. These aren't statistical noise. These are massive disparities in fundamental health outcomes—

and they exist despite the fact that we spend more than twice as much per person as the countries that are keeping their people healthier and alive longer.

So where does all that money go?

Administrative costs are a huge part of the answer. In 2017, the U.S. spent $812 billion on healthcare administration—$2,497 per capita, or 34.2% of all national health expenditures. That includes billing, insurance paperwork, prior authorizations, claims processing, all the bureaucratic machinery required to maintain our fragmented system. In comparison, Canada spends $551 per capita on healthcare administration—17% of expenditures. This means that we spend more than four times as much per person just shuffling papers and fighting with insurance companies.

The difference shows up in absurd places. Processing a single inpatient surgical bill costs $6 in Canada. In the United States, it costs $215.

We spend more on the administrative costs of healthcare than most countries spend on healthcare itself.

Drug prices are another piece. Americans pay the highest pharmaceutical prices in the world—roughly three times what other countries pay. Per capita pharmaceutical spending is $1,443 in the U.S. versus $466 to $939 in other high-income countries. Cancer drug prices in the U.S. are 2.02 to 2.42 times higher than in European countries. Americans are subsidizing pharmaceutical company profits that other countries refuse to pay.

But here's the thing that should make you furious: we don't get better care for all that extra spending. We get worse care, delivered less efficiently, with worse outcomes, at vastly higher cost.

A 2021 analysis by the Commonwealth Fund ranked the U.S. healthcare system last among eleven high-income countries across five domains: access to care, care process, administrative efficiency, equity, and health outcomes. Dead last. Behind the United Kingdom, Australia, the Netherlands, Germany, New Zealand, Sweden, France, Switzerland, Canada, and Norway.

The U.S. has ranked last in this comparison in 2004, 2006, 2007, 2010, and 2021. This isn't a fluke. It's not a temporary problem. It's systematic failure across decades.

We spend the most. We rank the worst.

This isn't a complicated mystery. Other countries have figured out how to deliver healthcare to their entire populations at half the cost with better results. They made different choices—policy choices, structural choices, values choices. They decided healthcare was a right, not a privilege. They built systems designed to keep people healthy rather than systems designed to extract maximum profit from people when they get sick.

We could have done the same thing. We still could.

First though, we'd have to be willing to ask an uncomfortable question: why didn't we?

And that's where the story gets ugly. Because the answer isn't about economics or efficiency or freedom or any of the other explanations you've been told. The answer is about who the system was designed to serve—and who it was designed to exclude.

So why does America have the healthcare system we have?

The answer isn't complicated, but it is uncomfortable: because the American healthcare system was deliberately designed to avoid being universal. It was designed that way because universal healthcare meant integration—and integration meant redistributing resources to Black Americans.

The Original Exclusion

The foundation of America's fragmented healthcare system was laid in 1935, long before most people think about when modern healthcare began. The Social Security Act of 1935—one of the landmark achievements of the New Deal—created the framework for employment-based benefits that still dominates American life today.

But it had a problem: Southern Democrats wouldn't support it if it included everyone.

So it didn't.

The Social Security Act deliberately excluded agricultural workers and domestic servants—the two occupations that employed the majority of Black Americans in 1935. This wasn't an oversight. It wasn't an unfortunate gap in coverage that would be fixed later. It was an explicit compromise designed to secure Southern votes by ensuring that Social Security benefits wouldn't go to Black workers.

The exclusion was staggeringly effective. In 1935, approximately 65% of Black workers were employed in agriculture or domestic service. By excluding these occupations, the Social Security Act effectively excluded two-thirds of Black Americans from the emerging social safety net while covering most White workers.

This created a two-tier system from the very beginning: employment-based benefits for those who qualified (predominantly White workers in industrial jobs) and nothing for those who didn't (predominantly Black workers in agriculture and domestic service).

This wasn't just about Social Security checks. The structure established by the 1935 act—tying economic security and benefits to employment status, not citizenship—became the template for how America would handle everything else, including healthcare.

Making It Permanent

The employment-based insurance model that dominates American healthcare today solidified during World War II, but not because anyone thought it was a good idea. It happened by accident—and then became permanent through deliberate policy choices.

During WWII, the federal government imposed wage controls to prevent inflation. Companies couldn't offer higher salaries to attract workers, so they competed by offering benefits instead—including health insurance. The IRS ruled that employer-provided health insurance wouldn't count as taxable income, making it an even more attractive benefit.

After the war, this arrangement could have been temporary. Other countries used the postwar period to build national health systems—the United Kingdom created the NHS in 1948, Canada began developing its universal system in the 1950s and 1960s. The United States could have done the same.

We didn't.

Instead, Congress passed the Taft-Hartley Act in 1947, which explicitly made employer-provided health insurance a subject of collective bargaining. This locked in the employment-based system, tying healthcare access to union membership and employment status. The unions that won the best healthcare benefits? Predominantly White industrial unions. The workers left out? Predominantly Black workers in agriculture, domestic service, and low-wage service jobs that weren't unionized.

The employment-based system wasn't chosen because it was efficient or effective. It was chosen—or more accurately, allowed to persist—because it maintained the racial hierarchy established by the Social Security Act. Healthcare became a job benefit, not a right. So if your job didn't provide it, that was your problem.

Federal Funding for Segregation

In 1946, Congress passed the Hill-Burton Act, officially called the Hospital Survey and Construction Act. It was supposed to address a genuine problem: America needed more hospitals, particularly in rural areas that were medically underserved.

The Hill-Burton Act provided federal funds—taxpayer dollars—to build hospitals across the country. Between 1946 and 1975, it funded nearly one-third of all hospital construction projects in America.

It also explicitly allowed those hospitals to be racially segregated.

The law included a "separate but equal" provision that permitted hospitals receiving federal construction funds to maintain separate facilities for White and Black patients. This wasn't a bug in the legislation—it was a feature, included specifically to secure Southern support.

So federal tax dollars—including taxes paid by Black Americans—funded the construction of hospitals that were legally allowed to refuse to treat Black patients, or to treat them only in inferior, segregated facilities.

The Hill-Burton Act wasn't repealed until 1964, after the Civil Rights Act made segregation illegal. By then, however, the infrastructure was already built. The hospital systems were established. The patterns of resource distribution—well-funded hospitals in White neighborhoods, underfunded or nonexistent facilities in Black neighborhoods—were set in concrete and steel.

You can still see the effects today. The neighborhoods that were redlined in the 1930s and 1940s—predominantly Black neighborhoods where banks refused to make loans and the government refused to invest—are the same neighborhoods that lack hospitals, have fewer primary care clinics, and have worse health outcomes today. That's not coincidence. That's design, built into the infrastructure with federal funding.

The Medicare-Medicaid Split

By the 1960s, the inadequacy of America's employment-based healthcare system was impossible to ignore. Elderly Americans who retired lost their employer-provided insurance exactly when they needed healthcare most. Poor Americans had no access to coverage at all.

So in 1965, Congress passed Medicare and Medicaid.

But here's where the design choices become critical: they created two separate programs with fundamentally different structures.

Medicare was universal for its target population. Every American over 65 got it, regardless of income, regardless of race, regardless of which state they lived in. It was a federal program with federal standards and federal funding.

Medicaid was means-tested, state-controlled, and optional. It covered "the poor"—but states got to define who counted as poor, what benefits they'd receive, and how generous the coverage would be. Southern states immediately used this flexibility to create restrictive eligibility requirements that excluded as many people as possible—particularly Black Americans.

Why create two separate programs? Why not just make Medicare universal for everyone, or make Medicaid federal and consistent?

Because universality was politically toxic.

In the 1960s, just like in the 1930s and 1940s, "universal" meant integration. It meant Black Americans and White Americans in the same system, receiving the same benefits, with the same access. It meant redistribution—taking tax revenue from predominantly White, wealthy states and using it to fund healthcare for predominantly Black, poor Americans.

That was unacceptable to Southern Democrats, who held enough power in Congress to block any legislation they opposed.

So we got two programs instead of one. Medicare for seniors—a politically sympathetic group that included plenty of White voters and therefore could be universal. Medicaid for the poor—a politically vulnerable group disproportionately Black and therefore could be state-controlled, means-tested, and stigmatized.

This wasn't an accident. This was the design.

Why "Universal" Became Toxic

Understanding the racial history of American healthcare policy explains something that confuses many people: why the word "universal" itself became politically toxic in American healthcare debates.

In other countries, "universal healthcare" just means everyone is covered. It's a practical description of a system design.

In America, "universal" became code for integration and redistribution. It meant dismantling the fragmented system that allowed White Americans to have better access, better facilities, and better outcomes than Black Americans. It meant taking resources from predominantly White communities and using them to fund healthcare for predominantly Black communities.

Politicians didn't have to say this explicitly—though many did, in barely-coded language about "welfare queens" and "undeserving poor." The structure spoke for itself. Keep healthcare employment-based, and you maintain the existing hierarchy. Keep Medicaid state-controlled, and Southern states can restrict access however they want. Resist "universal" healthcare, and you resist integration.

The healthcare policy debates of the past century weren't just about economics or freedom or government efficiency, though those arguments were made constantly. They were about maintaining racial hierarchy through system design.

The Legacy We Inherited

Today, the American healthcare system is a Rube Goldberg machine of complexity: employer-based insurance for some, Medicare for seniors, Medicaid for some poor people (depending on which state they live in), ACA marketplace plans for people who don't qualify for anything else, Veterans Administration for former military, Indian Health Service for Native Americans, the Federal Employees Health Benefits Program for government workers and members of Congress—who, notably, have access to some of the best healthcare coverage in the country while voting against universal coverage for everyone else—and nothing at all for the millions who fall through the cracks.

This fragmentation isn't an unfortunate side effect of a system that evolved organically. It's the direct result of deliberate policy choices made to avoid creating a universal system—because universal meant integration, and integration was unacceptable.

The racist foundation of the American healthcare system disadvantaged Black Americans most directly and most severely. That was the point. The effect, however, was that the fragmented system created to maintain racial hierarchy ended up harming everyone.

When healthcare is tied to employment, everyone—regardless of race—becomes vulnerable to job loss, employer decisions, and company bankruptcies. When coverage varies by state, everyone—regardless of race—faces instability if they move or live near a border. When the system is designed to be complicated and bureaucratic, everyone—regardless of race—drowns in paperwork and fights with insurance companies.

The racism that shaped American healthcare policy created a system that's uniquely terrible by every measure: most expensive, least efficient, worst outcomes, most administrative waste. We spend more per capita than any other developed nation and get less for it.

Could we have built something different? Of course. Every other developed nation did.

But we would have had to be willing to build a universal system. In America, at the time, universal meant integration, which meant redistribution to Black Americans. The active politicking against building that system—more than cost, more than freedom, more than any other argument you've heard—is why we have the healthcare system we have today.

It was designed this way. It's working exactly as intended—for the people it was designed to serve.

The rest of us just have to live with it. Or die trying to afford it.

And if you try to leave? The system has handcuffs for that too.

CHAPTER 2

The Insurance Trap

This opening scenario is hypothetical constructed to illustrate a common reality.

Marcus loved his job as a graphic designer at a small marketing agency in Portland. Or at least, he used to. After five years, the work had become repetitive, the deadlines relentless, the client demands exhausting. When a former colleague offered him a chance to join a startup—more creative freedom, equity stake, genuine opportunity to build something—he wanted to say yes immediately.

He said no. Because he couldn't risk losing his health insurance.

Marcus has high blood pressure—hypertension. It's controlled with medication, but his doctor keeps increasing the dose. At his last appointment, she'd looked at his numbers with concern. "Your stress levels are making this harder to manage," she'd told him. "You need to find ways to reduce stress." But the thing causing his stress was the job. And leaving the job meant losing insurance. Without insurance, his blood pressure medications cost $180 per month. His quarterly cardiology visits are $400 each. Managing his hypertension costs about $4,500 annually before insurance. His current employer-sponsored plan covers most of it.

The startup couldn't offer health insurance for the first year—too small, too new, barely funded. Marcus could buy coverage on the ACA marketplace, but the premium would be $650 monthly for a bronze plan with a $7,500 deductible. That's $7,800 in premiums plus potentially $7,500 out-of-pocket before insurance covers anything—$15,300 a year, minimum.

He couldn't afford it. So he stayed—trapped in a job that was worsening the condition he needed insurance to treat. Watching someone else take the opportunity he'd earned. Handcuffed to his employer by a chronic condition that affects nearly half of American adults.

This is called "job lock." It's not a bug in the American healthcare system—it's a feature.

How We Built the Trap

The employment-based insurance model that dominates American healthcare today wasn't designed by policy experts or healthcare economists. It emerged by accident during World War II and became permanent because it served powerful interests—just not yours.

During WWII, the federal government froze wages to prevent wartime inflation. Companies competing for workers couldn't offer higher salaries, so they competed with benefits instead. Health insurance became a recruitment tool—a way to attract employees when you couldn't pay them more.

In 1943, the IRS ruled that employer-provided health insurance wouldn't count as taxable income. This made it even more attractive: companies could offer $1,000 worth of health insurance for less than it would cost to give employees $1,000 in salary, because the salary would be taxed and the insurance wouldn't.

After the war ended, this arrangement could have been temporary. The wage controls were lifted. The emergency was over. As I mentioned, other countries, like the UK and Canada, used the postwar period to build national health systems.

The United States could have done the same. We had the wealth, the infrastructure, the political will for massive social programs. We built the interstate highway system, expanded Social Security, and funded universal public education.

But we didn't build universal healthcare.

Instead, Congress passed the Taft-Hartley Act in 1947, which made employer-provided health insurance a mandatory subject of collective bargaining. This locked the employment-based system into place. Unions negotiated for better health benefits instead of fighting for universal coverage. The best healthcare went to workers with strong unions—predominantly White industrial workers. Everyone else was on their own.

The system wasn't chosen because it was efficient. It was allowed to persist because it maintained the existing hierarchy: good coverage for workers with power, nothing for workers without it.

The Vulnerability by Design

Here's what makes the employment-based system uniquely cruel: you lose your health insurance exactly when you're most vulnerable.

Lose your job? Lose your coverage. Get laid off during a recession when finding new work takes months? No insurance while you're looking. Company goes bankrupt? Your health coverage disappears along with your paycheck.

You can keep your insurance through COBRA—the Consolidated Omnibus Budget Reconciliation Act, passed in 1985 to let people maintain coverage after leaving a job. Sounds helpful, right?

Except COBRA requires you to pay the full premium yourself—the amount your employer was paying plus the amount you were paying, plus a 2% administrative fee. For family coverage, that's often over $2,000 per month.

The following COBRA costs are from real Americans who shared their premiums in online discussions about healthcare costs in early 2026:

One woman in North Carolina, facing job loss, looked at her COBRA options: $1,625 per month for medical and vision coverage for her and her spouse. "COBRA is a no brainer," she wrote, with bitter sarcasm. "If I could stay on it for longer than 18 months, I absolutely would."

Another family—parents with two kids on COBRA—pays $2,200 per month. That's $26,400 per year, just for premiums, not counting deductibles or out-of-pocket costs.

A family of four in a different state: $3,200 per month for COBRA. The father noted, grimly, that if they paid cash for healthcare instead of using insurance, they'd spend $5,000 to $10,000 per year total.

With insurance, they spend $38,400 in premiums alone, plus a $500 deductible and $2,000 out-of-pocket maximum.

COBRA isn't a safety net. It's a technicality—legally, you can keep your insurance, but practically, almost nobody can afford to. During the COVID-19 pandemic, when millions lost their jobs, enrollment in public programs increased substantially while COBRA enrollment remained minimal. People couldn't afford it, not when they'd just lost their income.

So most people who lose their jobs lose their health insurance. They go without coverage, skip preventive care, ration medications, pray nothing serious happens until they find another job with benefits. And if something does happen—if they get sick or injured while uninsured—they face catastrophic medical bills that can destroy them financially.

The Insurance Company Profit Model

Let's be clear about how health insurance companies make money: they collect premiums from you every month, and then they do everything possible to avoid paying for your healthcare.

This isn't cynicism. It's their business model.

Insurance companies are for-profit businesses (even the "nonprofit" ones operate with similar incentives). Their revenue comes from premiums. Their costs come from paying claims. The less they pay in claims, the more profit they keep.

The Affordable Care Act tried to limit this with the medical loss ratio requirement: insurers must spend at least 80% of premium revenue on actual medical care in the individual and small group markets, or 85% in the large group market. If they spend less, they have to rebate the difference to customers.

Let's think about what that means. The law requires insurers to spend 80-85% of your premiums on your healthcare. Which means they're legally allowed to keep 15-20% for administrative costs and profit—money they make by NOT providing healthcare.

Before the ACA passed, many insurers weren't even meeting that low bar. In 2010, only 44% of individual market insurers spent 80% of premiums on care. By 2011, after the requirement took effect, that increased to 63%—which means more than a third of insurers still needed to change their practices to comply with a rule requiring them to spend barely 80% of customers' money on actual healthcare.

But even after the ACA, insurance companies have countless ways to minimize what they pay out.

Deny, Delay, Defend

Remember those three words engraved on the bullet casings found after Brian Thompson's assassination? "Deny. Defend. Depose."

The shooter was referencing a book called *Delay, Deny, Defend* by law professor Jay Feinman, which documented how insurance companies systematically avoid paying legitimate claims. The strategy is simple and effective:

Deny the claim initially. Just say no. Many people won't appeal—they'll give up, pay out of pocket, or go without the care entirely.

Delay the ones who do appeal. Make them submit more paperwork. Request additional documentation. Require prior authorization. Make the process so exhausting and time-consuming that people give up or die waiting.

Defend aggressively if they make it to legal action. Spend whatever it takes on lawyers to avoid paying claims, knowing most individuals can't afford to match those legal resources.

In 2023, insurance companies denied 20% of claims in the ACA marketplace. One in five claims—denied. Fewer than 1% of denials were appealed, which means most people just accepted the denial and either paid out of pocket or went without care.

For Medicare Advantage plans—the private insurance version of Medicare—insurers made nearly 50 million prior authorization determinations in 2023. They denied 6.4% of them, and only 11.7% of denials were appealed.

These numbers sound small—6.4%, 20%—until you remember we're talking about millions of people. 20% of ACA marketplace claims means millions of denials. 6.4% of Medicare Advantage determinations means over three million denials.

And these are just the claims people bothered to file. The system is designed to discourage people from seeking care in the first place.

Prior Authorization: Bureaucracy as Obstacle

Prior authorization is theoretically a cost-control mechanism—insurers want to review expensive treatments before approving them to make sure they're medically necessary. In practice, it's a bureaucratic obstacle course designed to delay and deny care.

Your doctor orders an MRI. Before you can get it, your insurance company requires "prior authorization"—your doctor's office has to submit paperwork explaining why you need the MRI, including your symptoms, medical history, and why other diagnostic tests won't work. Then you wait.

And wait.

And wait.

Sometimes for days. Sometimes for weeks. Sometimes your insurance company denies the authorization, and your doctor has to appeal, submitting more paperwork, and you wait longer. Meanwhile, your symptoms continue. Your condition potentially worsens. Your anxiety builds.

Sometimes the prior authorization gets approved after you've already had the test—meaning you went through the bureaucratic process even though the outcome was guaranteed approval, just to create paperwork and delay.

Insurance companies know this. They know that making people jump through hoops discourages them from seeking care. They know that delays wear people down. They know that some people will give up rather than fight through the bureaucracy.

That's the point.

The Cost of Coverage

Let's talk about what people actually pay for health insurance in 2026—not theoretical numbers, but real premiums from real people.

The following are real premiums shared by real Americans in a January 2026 online discussion about healthcare costs. Names have been removed, but the numbers are exact as reported:

A 42-year-old single woman in Michigan: $409 per month for a bronze plan with a $7,500 deductible and $10,000 out-of-pocket maximum. That's $4,908 per year in premiums, and she has to spend another $7,500 before insurance pays anything beyond preventive care.

A woman in Florida, bronze plan, high deductible: $1,130 per month with a $6,500 deductible and $7,500 out-of-pocket maximum. She's already hit that maximum this year because she was diagnosed with breast cancer. So she'll pay $13,560 in premiums plus $7,500 out of pocket—$21,060 total. For a single person. With insurance.

A couple in Florida paying $2,535 per month—$30,420 per year—with a $6,700 deductible per person and $7,400 maximum out-of-pocket. Their premium increased from $1,800 per month the previous year when Aetna pulled out of Florida, reducing their options.

A family in Washington, DC, bronze HSA plan: $660 per month premium, $6,350 annual deductible, $7,300 out-of-pocket maximum. That's the "most affordable" plan they could find.

A couple with a child, bronze plan: $344 per month. Sounds reasonable, except the husband is an independent contractor who can't get insurance any other way, and they're paying that on reduced income.

A person in rural North Carolina noted that premiums went up over 40% from 2025 to 2026. "It's nuts to pay $1,000/month for a bronze plan and still have to meet a deductible for anything except preventative visits," they wrote.

And here's the thing that keeps coming up: geography matters as much as anything else. One person noted that living in a rural county with poor health rankings meant their premiums would be $200-300 less per month if they lived one county west, with more options available.

Some counties have only two or three insurance options. Some have only one. There's no federal mandate requiring insurers to offer plans anywhere—if a county seems too risky or not profitable enough, insurers just pull out, leaving residents with limited choices or no choices at all.

This is what the "free market" in healthcare looks like. You pay thousands of dollars per year for the privilege of having insurance, and then you pay thousands more before that insurance actually covers anything. If you live in the wrong county or have the wrong medical history or work for the wrong employer, your options are even worse.

Why Employers Hate This Too

Here's something that rarely gets discussed: employers don't actually want to provide health insurance.

It's expensive. It's complicated. It creates an enormous administrative burden. HR departments spend countless hours negotiating with insurance companies, managing enrollment, handling employee complaints about coverage denials and network limitations.

Small businesses especially struggle with this. A company with 10 employees can't negotiate the same rates as a company with 10,000 employees. They pay higher premiums for worse coverage, making it harder to compete for talent against larger companies.

Every year, employers face brutal decisions: raise premiums for employees, reduce coverage, increase deductibles, or absorb higher costs themselves and accept lower profits. There are no good options.

Many businesses would happily get out of the healthcare business entirely—if there were somewhere else for their employees to get coverage. There just isn't. So they're stuck providing insurance because that's what employees need to survive, and employees are stuck with employer-provided insurance because there's no viable alternative.

Everyone is trapped in a system that serves almost no one's interests—except insurance companies, who profit from the complexity, and politicians, who take campaign donations from the insurance industry to keep it this way.

The Trap Today

The employment-based healthcare system creates cascading vulnerabilities that affect everyone differently but harm almost everyone:

You're trapped by your job. You can't leave for a better opportunity. You can't start a business. You can't retire early. You can't take time off to care for a sick family member or recover from your own illness. Your healthcare coverage controls your life choices in ways that have nothing to do with your health or your career.

Your employer is trapped providing coverage. They'd rather spend money on wages, research and development, business growth—anything except negotiating with insurance companies. Simultaneously, they can't compete for employees without offering health benefits, so they're stuck.

Insurance companies profit from the complexity. The more

confusing the system, the more people give up on appealing denials. The more bureaucratic the process, the more people avoid seeking care. The more fragmented the market, the less negotiating power anyone has. Complexity is profitable—for insurers.

Politicians maintain the system. Insurance and pharmaceutical companies are among the biggest political donors in America. They fund campaigns, hire lobbyists, and fight viciously against any proposal for universal healthcare. And politicians who benefit from those donations have no incentive to change a system that works perfectly well—for their donors.

Everyone else just has to live with it. Or die trying to afford it.

The employment-based insurance system isn't a natural feature of healthcare. It's not the inevitable result of free-market forces, American values, or economic necessity. It's a historical accident that became permanent through deliberate policy choices, maintained by industries that profit from it, and justified by politicians who benefit from campaign donations.

We chose this system. We could choose differently.

But first, we'd have to acknowledge that the trap isn't a bug—it's part of the system's design. A system whose main beneficiaries are the companies that provide the products we all rely on for quality of life, health, and even survival.

CHAPTER 3

Big Pharma's Rise

This opening scenario is hypothetical, constructed to illustrate a common reality.

Nicole woke up at 3 a.m. feeling wrong. Not sick, exactly—just off. Her mouth was dry. She was thirsty but also nauseous. Her heart was racing.

She knew what was happening. She'd been rationing her insulin again.

Nicole has Type 1 diabetes. Her body doesn't produce insulin, so she has to inject it multiple times per day to stay alive. Without insulin, glucose builds up in her blood, and her body starts breaking down fat for energy instead. This produces ketones, which make the blood acidic. It's called diabetic ketoacidosis (DKA), and it will kill you.

She'd been stretching her insulin for three weeks, taking slightly less than prescribed to make the vial last longer. The math was simple: her prescription called for two vials per month. With insurance, each vial cost her $99. Without insurance—which she'd lost when her hours got cut at work—the cash price was $340 per vial.

She couldn't afford $680 a month. So she rationed.

By 4 a.m., Nicole was vomiting. By 6 a.m., her roommate found her unconscious and called 911. The ER stabilized her, gave her IV insulin and fluids, kept her for observation. The bill was $8,400. She had no insurance and no way to pay it.

Nicole survived. Many don't.

Between 2017 and 2019, at least 1.3 million Americans with diabetes rationed insulin due to cost. The exact number who died isn't tracked—those deaths get classified as "diabetic complications" rather than what they actually are: deaths from inability to afford medication.

Here's what makes Nicole's story particularly obscene: insulin was discovered in 1921, over a century ago. The researchers who discovered it sold the patent to the University of Toronto for $1, believing it was too important to restrict with profit motives. It costs approximately $10 to manufacture a vial of insulin.

Nicole was paying $340 for something that costs $10 to make.

That's not healthcare. That's predatory capitalism wearing a white coat.

This predatory practice is not unique to insulin. It's how the entire pharmaceutical industry operates in America.

From Healing to Profit

Pharmaceutical companies didn't always work this way.

In the mid-20th century, drug companies were research institutions that also made money, rather than profit machines that also did research. Scientists ran them. The focus was on discovering new treatments, solving medical problems, advancing human health. Profit mattered, but it wasn't the only thing that mattered.

That changed in the 1980s and 1990s.

Wall Street discovered pharmaceuticals. Finance executives replaced scientists in the C-suite. Shareholder value became the primary—often the only—metric of success. Marketing budgets exploded, exceeding research and development spending. Companies stopped asking "What disease can we cure?" and started asking "What price can we charge?"

The shift was dramatic and deliberate. CEOs with finance backgrounds took over. Stock price became more important than patient outcomes. Quarterly earnings reports mattered more than long-term research. The entire industry reoriented around a single question: How do we maximize profit?

The answer, it turned out, was simple: charge as much as people will pay before they die.

"Orphan drugs"—medications for rare diseases—became particularly lucrative. Small patient populations meant less price resistance. Desperate patients meant higher willingness to pay. Limited competition meant monopoly pricing. Companies started buying rights to old, cheap drugs and jacking up prices overnight.

This wasn't about funding research. This was about extracting maximum profit from human suffering.

The Price Gouging Playbook

In 2022, the FDA approved Hemgenix, a gene therapy treatment for hemophilia B. The price: $3.5 million per treatment.

$3.5 million dollars. For a single treatment.

The company, CSL Behring, justified this price by arguing the treatment is one-time and potentially curative, eliminating the need for ongoing factor replacement therapy. They framed $3.5 million as a bargain compared to lifetime treatment costs.

Here's the thing, though: we have no idea what Hemgenix actually costs to manufacture. The company won't say. We know the research was largely publicly funded through NIH grants. We know gene therapy manufacturing has gotten dramatically cheaper as the technology has scaled. But the pricing isn't based on costs plus reasonable profit—it's based on "what the market will bear."

In healthcare, "what the market will bear" means "how much can we charge before you die or go bankrupt?"

Hemgenix is an extreme example, but the pattern is universal. American patients pay wildly more for medications than patients in any other developed country—for the exact same drugs, made by the exact same companies, with the same ingredients and the same manufacturing processes.

After accounting for purchasing power parity, U.S. drug prices are three times higher than Germany's. The U.S. price index sits at 298.2 compared to Germany's baseline of 100. For some medications, Americans pay ten, twenty, even thirty times what patients in other countries pay.

Why?

Not because American drugs are better. Not because manufacturing costs are higher here. Not because research is more expensive.

Because American law allows pharmaceutical companies to charge whatever they want.

In 2003, Congress passed the Medicare Modernization Act, which created Medicare Part D prescription drug coverage. Buried in that legislation was a provision that explicitly prohibited Medicare from negotiating drug prices with pharmaceutical companies.

Let that sink in.

Medicare covers prescription drugs for approximately 40 million Americans—29% of the nation's total prescription drug expenditure. The federal government is the single largest purchaser of pharmaceuticals in America. And Congress made it *illegal* for Medicare to negotiate prices.

Every other aspect of Medicare involves negotiation or set prices. The government negotiates hospital rates. It sets reimbursement schedules for procedures. But for drugs? No negotiation allowed. Pharmaceutical companies can charge *whatever they want*, and Medicare *has to pay it*.

This wasn't an accident. This was deliberate policy, bought and paid for by pharmaceutical industry lobbying.

From 1999 to 2018, the pharmaceutical and health product industry spent $4.7 billion on federal lobbying—an average of $233 million per year, more than any other industry. The Pharmaceutical Research and Manufacturers of America (PhRMA) alone accounted for $422 million of that spending.

They also spent $414 million on campaign contributions to presidential and congressional candidates. Of the 20 senators and 20 representatives who received the most pharmaceutical industry contributions, 39 served on committees with jurisdiction over health-related legislation, with 24 in senior leadership positions.

That's not influence. That's purchase.

The result? Americans pay obscene prices for medications while pharmaceutical executives get rich and shareholders profit from human suffering.

In 2016, Mylan increased the price of EpiPens—lifesaving devices for people with severe allergies—from around $100 to over $600. The medication inside hadn't changed. The device hadn't improved. The manufacturing costs were essentially identical. Mylan just decided they could charge more, so they did.

In 2015, Martin Shkreli's company Turing Pharmaceuticals bought the rights to Daraprim, a drug used to treat parasitic infections in immunocompromised patients. Overnight, they raised the price from $13.50 per pill to $750—a 5,000% increase. Same drug. Same formulation. No improvements. Just pure price gouging.

These weren't isolated incidents. They're how the system works.

Patent Evergreening

Pharmaceutical patents are supposed to work like this: a company develops a new drug, gets a patent that gives them exclusive rights to manufacture it for 20 years, charges premium prices during that period to recoup research costs and make profit, and then the patent expires and generic manufacturers can make cheaper versions.

That's the theory. Here's the reality.

Pharmaceutical companies have become experts at "evergreening"—gaming the patent system to extend their monopoly far beyond 20 years. They make minor modifications to existing drugs and claim them as new inventions worthy of new patents. A new delivery mechanism. A slightly different dosage. A time-release formulation. An extended-release version.

These aren't meaningful improvements. They're strategic tweaks designed solely to block generic competition.

AbbVie's Humira, a drug for autoimmune conditions, accumulated over 100 patents—not because the drug kept getting dramatically better, but because AbbVie kept making minor modifications and claiming each one deserved patent protection. This "patent thicket" strategy successfully blocked generic competition for years beyond the original patent expiration, allowing AbbVie to continue charging premium prices.

Companies also engage in "pay-for-delay" deals, where brand-name manufacturers pay generic companies to delay bringing competing products to market. Legally, this is supposed to be prohibited as anticompetitive. In practice, pharmaceutical companies structure these agreements carefully enough to avoid prosecution while achieving the same result: delayed competition, extended monopoly pricing, continued profit extraction.

The cost to patients? Billions of dollars annually in overpriced medications that should have generic alternatives available.

The Opioid Epidemic

In 1996, Purdue Pharma launched OxyContin with the most aggressive pharmaceutical marketing campaign in American history.

They didn't just advertise to doctors—they created an entire ecosystem designed to maximize opioid prescriptions. They promoted the idea of "pain as the fifth vital sign," encouraging doctors to treat any reported pain aggressively. They funded pain advocacy groups that pushed for expanded opioid use. They embedded pro-opioid messaging in international medical guidance documents. They cultivated close relationships with U.S. elected officials.

They also lied. Systematically, deliberately, catastrophically.

Purdue marketed OxyContin as having less than 1% addiction risk—a completely fabricated statistic with no scientific basis. They trained sales representatives to downplay addiction risks and emphasize the drug's safety. They targeted states without triplicate prescription programs—regulatory safeguards that required special paperwork for controlled substances—because those states had less oversight.

The strategy worked. OxyContin distribution was more than 50% lower in states with triplicate programs. States without those protections experienced substantially faster growth in overdose deaths—growth that continued for over 20 years after OxyContin's launch.

Purdue knew what they were doing. Internal documents later revealed that executives were aware of widespread abuse, diversion, and addiction. They knew doctors were overprescribing. They knew patients were becoming addicted. They knew people were dying.

They didn't stop. They doubled down.

Sales representatives received bonuses for getting doctors to prescribe higher doses and longer-duration prescriptions—exactly the prescribing patterns most likely to cause addiction. Purdue specifically targeted rural communities and Appalachia, areas with limited healthcare infrastructure and populations vulnerable to exploitation.

The result: over 600,000 deaths in North America from the opioid epidemic that Purdue Pharma deliberately created and sustained for profit.

In 2007, Purdue Pharma and three executives pleaded guilty to federal charges of misbranding OxyContin. The company paid $600 million in fines. The executives paid $34.5 million personally. None went to prison.

The Sackler family, which owned Purdue Pharma, extracted billions of dollars from the company before declaring bankruptcy. They used complex financial maneuvers to shield their personal wealth. When Purdue finally filed for bankruptcy in 2019, the Sacklers negotiated a settlement that allowed them to keep most of their fortune in exchange for contributing to opioid treatment programs.

They killed hundreds of thousands of people, made billions of dollars doing it, and faced virtually no personal consequences.

This isn't ancient history. This happened in the 1990s and 2000s.

Many of the executives involved are still alive, still wealthy, still living comfortable lives while the families of their victims buried their dead.

That's American pharmaceutical regulation in action.

The Insulin Scandal

Let's return to insulin—the drug discovered over a century ago, given to the world with the hope it would save lives affordably.

Three companies control approximately 90% of the global insulin market: Eli Lilly, Novo Nordisk, and Sanofi. Between 1996 and 2019, they increased insulin prices by 1,200%.

Not because insulin got better. The formulations didn't fundamentally change. Manufacturing didn't get dramatically more expensive. Research costs didn't suddenly spike.

The prices went up because the companies could raise them—and because they raised them together, in a pattern called "shadow pricing." When one company increased prices, the others matched. They moved in lockstep, eliminating any competitive pressure to keep prices reasonable.

The result? Americans with Type 1 diabetes—who need insulin to survive—faced impossible choices. Some rationed their insulin, taking less than prescribed to make it last longer. Some skipped doses entirely. Some bought insulin from Canada or Mexico, where the exact same products cost a fraction of U.S. prices. Some bought older, less effective formulations from Walmart because they were marginally cheaper.

Some died.

Between 2017 and 2019, at least 1.3 million Americans with diabetes rationed insulin due to cost. We don't know exactly how many died—those deaths get classified as diabetes complications, not as what they actually are: preventable deaths caused by inability to afford medication.

The companies knew this was happening. They had the data. They saw the reports. They knew people were dying because insulin cost too much.

They kept raising prices anyway.

In 2022, the Inflation Reduction Act finally capped insulin costs at $35 per month—but only for Medicare recipients. If you're under the age of 65 and not on Medicare, you can still pay hundreds of dollars per month for a drug that costs $10 to manufacture.

The fact that the government can cap insulin prices for Medicare patients proves it can do so for everyone. The fact that they haven't—that insulin remains unaffordable for millions of Americans—isn't about economics or feasibility.

It's about politics, lobbying, campaign contributions—and the fundamental decision to let the pharmaceutical companies' profits matter more than human lives.

Why This Only Happens in America

Every other developed nation negotiates pharmaceutical prices.

Canada has the Patented Medicine Prices Review Board, which sets maximum prices for new drugs based on comparison to international prices and therapeutic benefit. If a price seems excessive, the board can require reductions or rebates.

The United Kingdom has the National Institute for Health and Care Excellence (NICE), which evaluates whether new drugs provide enough benefit to justify their cost. If NICE determines a drug isn't cost-effective, the National Health Service won't cover it—which means the pharmaceutical company either lowers the price or loses access to the UK market.

Germany, France, Japan, Australia—every developed nation has some mechanism for controlling drug prices through negotiation, price review boards, or cost-effectiveness analysis.

The result? The same drugs Americans pay hundreds or thousands of dollars for cost a fraction of that price everywhere else.

Pharmaceutical companies justify U.S. prices by claiming they need the revenue to fund research and development. "Americans pay more because we're funding innovation for the world," they argue. "If we cap prices, pharmaceutical research will collapse and new drugs will stop being developed."

This is a lie.

From 2010 to 2019, the National Institutes of Health funded research that contributed to 354 of 356 drugs approved by the FDA—99.4% of new drugs.

Total NIH investment: $187 billion.

But here's the critical detail: only 3.3% of that NIH funding—$8.1 billion—went to phased clinical trials, the formal development pathway required for FDA approval. The vast majority, 84.9%, funded basic research on biological targets.

In other words, American taxpayers fund the basic science that makes new drugs possible. Pharmaceutical companies take that publicly funded research, develop it into marketable products, and then charge Americans premium prices for drugs that wouldn't exist without public investment.

For first-to-target drugs—meaning truly novel medications rather than variations on existing treatments—NIH spending exceeded reported industry spending by nearly $2 billion. We're not just subsidizing pharmaceutical research. We're often doing more of it than the companies themselves.

The argument that high U.S. prices fund global innovation is propaganda designed to justify price gouging. American patients are subsidizing lower prices worldwide, unable to afford medications developed with their own tax dollars, while pharmaceutical executives get rich claiming they're heroes of innovation.

The Political Protection

The pharmaceutical industry doesn't just charge whatever they want. They've built a political fortress to protect their ability to do so.

PhRMA—the Pharmaceutical Research and Manufacturers of America—is one of the most powerful lobbying organizations in Washington. From 1999 to 2018, they spent $422 million on federal lobbying. The broader pharmaceutical and health product industry spent $4.7 billion over the same period—$233 million per year on average, more than any other industry.

They also spent $414 million on campaign contributions during that time. The money went to both parties, to presidential candidates and congressional races, to national party committees and outside spending groups. Of the 40 members of Congress who received the most pharmaceutical industry contributions, 39 served on committees with jurisdiction over health-related legislation.

This isn't influence. This is institutional capture.

The result is a revolving door between pharmaceutical companies and regulatory agencies. FDA officials leave to become pharmaceutical executives. Pharmaceutical executives join the FDA in senior positions. Congressional staffers who work on healthcare policy get hired by pharmaceutical companies as lobbyists and consultants.

Every attempt at meaningful pharmaceutical price reform gets crushed.

The Medicare Part D negotiation ban—the provision that prohibited Medicare from negotiating drug prices—was included specifically because pharmaceutical companies lobbied for it. They argued that government negotiating power would decrease industry revenues and therefore decrease research and development. Congress bought the argument (or rather, was paid to buy the argument) and prohibited negotiation for Medicare's prescription drug benefit.

This prohibition remained in place for nearly 20 years, costing Medicare—and therefore taxpayers—hundreds of billions of dollars in overpayments.

President Trump promised repeatedly to lower drug prices. "We're going to bring down prescription drug prices," he said in 2017. "We're going to bring them way down." He promised to allow reimportation of drugs from Canada. He promised to end the practice of charging Americans more than other countries. He promised to take on pharmaceutical companies.

He accomplished essentially none of it. Pharmaceutical lobbying and campaign contributions ensured that meaningful reform never happened.

President Biden's Inflation Reduction Act (IRA), passed in 2022, finally allowed limited Medicare drug price negotiation. The first 10 drugs were selected in August 2023, with negotiated prices taking effect in 2026. The program scales up to 60 drugs by 2029, with Part B drugs not included until 2028 [Medicare Part B covers only drugs that are not usually self-administered].

This is genuine progress—simulations suggest it could have saved $26.5 billion from 2018 to 2020, and the Congressional Budget Office estimated $100 billion in savings from 2022 to 2031.

But here's the reality: the first round of negotiations achieved only 22% average price reduction—less than half of initial projections. Furthermore, the program is already being weakened. The One Big Beautiful Bill Act of 2025 expanded orphan drug exclusions, delaying eligibility for 5 products and excluding at least 3 from future negotiations entirely.

Even when negotiation happens, it's pathetically limited. Drugs must have been on the market for at least 9 years (13 for biologics), can't have generic competitors, and must exceed $200 million in annual Medicare spending. The maximum negotiated price is still 40-75% of the manufacturer's price—which means "negotiated" prices can remain exorbitant.

Pharmaceutical companies are already gaming it. They're raising launch prices by an estimated 11% for Part D drugs and 2% for Part B drugs to compensate for future negotiations.

The projected savings? About 1.1% of Medicare spending—modest relative to the $806 billion Americans spent on prescription drugs in 2024.

Translation: Medicare can negotiate drug prices, but only for a handful of drugs, only after they've been overpriced for nearly a decade, only within limits that still allow pharmaceutical companies to charge obscene amounts, and companies are already finding workarounds.

This isn't reform—it's theater designed to look like reform while protecting pharmaceutical profits.

And pharmaceutical companies are suing to block even this modest reform, arguing that price negotiation violates their constitutional rights.

They're not wrong to fight it. The IRA threatens their business model. If Americans start paying reasonable prices for medications, pharmaceutical company profits will decrease. Stock prices might fall. Executive bonuses might shrink.

From their perspective, that's unacceptable. Better to let Americans die bankrupt than accept slightly lower profit margins.

The Design

The American pharmaceutical system isn't broken. It's working exactly as intended—for pharmaceutical companies, their shareholders, and the politicians they fund.

For everyone else, it's a predatory nightmare.

We pay the highest drug prices in the world for medications developed with our own tax dollars. We ration lifesaving treatments because we can't afford them. We die from preventable causes while pharmaceutical executives vacation in the Hamptons on bonuses extracted from our suffering.

This isn't healthcare. This is extraction.

It will continue until we decide that human lives matter more than pharmaceutical industry profits—and until we elect politicians willing to say so even when it costs them campaign contributions.

> *First, though, we will have to take a long, hard look at what in our model allows people to become so sick that long-term care is their only option.*

PART 2

THE CURRENT CRISIS

CHAPTER 4

The Reactive Model

This opening scenario is hypothetical, constructed to illustrate a common reality.

David was 52 when his doctor told him his cholesterol was high. Not dangerously high—just elevated. LDL at 160, when it should be under 100. His doctor recommended lifestyle changes: better diet, more exercise, maybe a low-dose statin if the numbers didn't improve within six months.

David didn't have health insurance. He'd been working as an independent contractor for three years, and the cheapest marketplace plan he could find cost $650 a month with a $7,500 deductible. He couldn't afford it, so he went without.

The follow-up appointment his doctor recommended? $400 out of pocket. The statin prescription if he needed it? About $30 a month for the generic. The quarterly monitoring to make sure the medication wasn't causing liver problems? Another $200 each time.

David did the math. He was feeling fine. High cholesterol doesn't hurt—there are no symptoms, no warning signs, no immediate consequences. So he skipped the follow-up. Figured he'd eat better, exercise more, deal with it when he could afford to.

Two years later, David had a stroke.

He woke up one morning unable to move his right arm. His face drooped on one side. When he tried to call for help, the words came out slurred and wrong. His neighbor found him three hours later and called 911.

The ambulance ride cost $2,400. The emergency room visit, CT scan, and initial treatment cost $18,000. Five days in the hospital for monitoring and rehabilitation: $47,000. Follow-up care, medications, physical therapy to regain function in his arm: another $30,000 over six months.

Total: approximately $97,400 to treat a stroke that could have been prevented with $30-a-month medication and a few hundred dollars in monitoring.

David survived, but he never fully recovered. His right hand doesn't work well enough to do his old job. He's on permanent disability now, which finally qualified him for Medicaid. The system ignored him when prevention was cheap. It engaged when treatment became catastrophically expensive.

This isn't a failure of the American healthcare system. This is exactly how it's designed to work.

Why Prevention Doesn't Pay

The financial incentives in American healthcare are backwards. The system doesn't profit from keeping you healthy—it profits from treating you when you get sick.

Prevention pays once. You screen for cancer, find it early, treat it successfully—that's one round of revenue. You vaccinate a child against measles—that's one payment, and then that child never generates revenue from measles treatment. You help someone with prediabetes change their diet and exercise habits so they never develop diabetes—you've just eliminated decades of potential revenue from diabetes management.

Disease management, on the other hand, pays forever.

A patient with Type 2 diabetes generates revenue for 20, 30, 40 years. Medications, test strips, glucose monitors, quarterly check-ups, annual eye exams, foot exams, kidney function tests. As the disease progresses—and it often does, because the system isn't designed to help people reverse it—the revenue increases. Neuropathy treatments. Cardiovascular medications. Eventually dialysis, at $90,000 per year. Possibly amputations. Hospital admissions for complications.

From a business perspective, preventing diabetes is terrible. Managing diabetes is a gold mine.

The cost-effectiveness data proves this backwards incentive structure. Diabetes prevention programs—lifestyle interventions helping people with prediabetes avoid developing full diabetes—cost approximately $12,510 per quality-adjusted life year (QALY). That's well below the $50,000 threshold generally considered cost-effective in healthcare.

Metformin, a cheap generic medication that can prevent diabetes in high-risk patients, costs even less: $17,089 per QALY. Studies of the National Diabetes Prevention Program show an 88% probability of actually saving money over just two years, with an average reduction of $4,552 in direct medical costs per enrollee.

Prevention doesn't just work—it saves money.

Here's the problem with preventive care: the savings accrue to society, to the healthcare system as a whole, to future insurers. The entity paying for prevention today often doesn't benefit from the prevention working 5 or 10 years from now, because the patient will likely have different insurance by then.

So prevention gets ignored, underfunded, deprioritized. As a result, patients like David end up having strokes that cost $100,000 to treat instead of spending $2,000 over two years to prevent.

The Chronic Disease Gold Mine

Let's follow the money through a typical chronic disease progression and see why the system prefers sick patients to healthy ones.

Stage 1: Prediabetes. Blood sugar is elevated but not quite diabetic. This is the prevention window. Lifestyle intervention—dietary changes, exercise programs, behavioral support—can reverse prediabetes and prevent diabetes from developing.

Cost: approximately $400-$600 per person for a structured prevention program.

Revenue to the healthcare system: minimal. Maybe one or two doctor visits per year for monitoring. No medications yet. No complications. From a profit perspective, this patient is almost worthless.

Stage 2: Type 2 Diabetes, newly diagnosed. Now the patient needs medication—metformin to start, maybe other drugs as the disease progresses. Quarterly doctor visits. Regular lab work. Annual eye exams and foot exams. Test strips and glucose monitors.

Revenue: substantially higher. A conservative estimate would be \$3,000-\$5,000 per year. The patient will likely have this disease for 20-40 years. That's \$60,000 to \$200,000 in lifetime revenue, and we're just getting started.

Stage 3: Complications. After 10-15 years of diabetes, complications often develop. Cardiovascular disease—the leading cause of death in diabetics. Kidney disease. Neuropathy. Retinopathy that can lead to blindness.

Now the patient needs more medications: statins for cholesterol, blood pressure medications, medications for neuropathy pain. More specialist visits—cardiologist, nephrologist, ophthalmologist. More procedures—cardiac catheterizations, possibly stents or bypass surgery.

Revenue: \$15,000-\$30,000 per year, easily. This continues for the rest of the patient's life.

Stage 4: End-stage complications. Kidney failure requiring dialysis. Amputations from neuropathy and poor circulation. Heart failure requiring repeated hospitalizations.

Dialysis alone costs approximately \$90,000 per year. Hospital admissions for heart failure: \$15,000-\$30,000 per admission, and patients often have multiple admissions per year.

Revenue: \$100,000+ annually. For a disease that could have been prevented at Stage 1 for $500.

This progression isn't inevitable. Diabetes can be managed well, complications can be delayed or prevented, some people even reverse Type 2 diabetes through significant lifestyle changes. But the system isn't designed to help people do that. It's designed to manage the disease and treat the complications—because that's where the money is.

The same pattern holds for cardiovascular disease. High blood pressure, if caught early and treated with generic medication and lifestyle changes, costs maybe $1,000-$2,000 per year to manage. If it's allowed to progress, however—atherosclerosis, heart attack, stents, bypass surgery, heart failure—the revenue skyrockets. A single cardiac catheterization with stent placement can cost $30,000-$50,000. Bypass surgery: $70,000-$200,000. Then the patient will require ongoing management of heart failure for the rest of their life.

Cancer screening versus cancer treatment shows the same economics. A colonoscopy costs $1,000-$3,000. If it finds a polyp early, removal is simple and cheap. But if that polyp progresses to colon cancer? Stage 3 colon cancer treatment—surgery, chemotherapy, radiation, follow-up care—can cost $200,000 to $500,000.

Multicomponent interventions to increase colorectal cancer screening are actually cost-saving—they save more money than they cost by catching cancer early. Despite this, screening programs remain underfunded and underutilized, because the insurance company paying for screening today won't necessarily be the one paying for cancer treatment 10 years from now.

In short, the system incentivizes the $500,000 cancer treatment, not the $3,000 colonoscopy that would prevent it.

What Prevention Actually Costs vs. Returns

The return on investment for preventive care is staggering—if you measure it honestly.

Childhood vaccinations prevent diseases that would cost millions to treat if they occurred at pre-vaccine rates. The measles, mumps, and rubella (MMR) vaccine costs about $70. A single case of measles requiring hospitalization can cost $50,000-$100,000. Before the measles vaccine, the U.S. had hundreds of thousands of cases annually. The vaccine essentially eliminated the disease in America.

We're bringing it back.

As of May 2025, over 1,000 measles cases and 3 deaths have been reported—the highest numbers in more than 25 years. 96% of cases involved unvaccinated individuals. MMR vaccination coverage has fallen below 95% in nearly two-thirds of U.S. counties—the threshold needed for herd immunity.

At current vaccination rates, measles will likely become endemic again within two decades. If vaccination rates decline by 50%—a scenario actively being debated in policy circles—we're looking at 51 million measles cases, 10 million hospitalizations, and 159,000 deaths over 25 years.

Let that sink in: 159,000 deaths. From a disease we've already eliminated once.

The economics haven't changed. Routine childhood vaccination among children born 1994-2023 prevented 508 million cases of illness, 32 million hospitalizations, and 1.1 million deaths, saving $540 billion in direct costs and $2.7 trillion in societal costs. For every dollar spent on childhood vaccines, society saves $7.50.

However, these savings only materialize if children get vaccinated, and vaccination rates are collapsing.

Less than 70% of U.S. children now receive the full series of recommended vaccinations by 24 months. Non-medical exemptions are increasing. Policy debates are questioning routine vaccine recommendations and considering removal of school-based vaccine mandates.

This isn't happening because vaccines stopped working. It's happening because prevention doesn't generate profit the way treatment does. Vaccinating a child costs $70. Treating measles complications generates tens of thousands in hospital revenue. The reactive model rewards letting children get sick and then charging their families to save them.

HPV vaccination combined with cervical cancer screening costs $86 to $476 per quality-adjusted life year gained. Cervical cancer treatment costs $50,000-$200,000. Screening interventions cost $159 per additional woman screened—and prevent cancers that would bankrupt families to treat.

The math is obvious. Prevention is cheaper and more effective, but the system doesn't reward preventing disease—it rewards treating disease after it's already caused suffering.

We're dismantling one of public health's greatest achievements not because it stopped working, but because it works too well. Healthy children don't generate healthcare revenue. Sick children do.

The consequences are already here: over 1,000 measles cases in 2025 after years of near-elimination, with modeling predicting endemic measles within two decades. Again: we eliminated this disease. We're choosing to bring it back.

That's the reactive model in action.

Breast cancer screening interventions cost about $148 per additional woman screened. Catching breast cancer at Stage 1 versus Stage 3 can mean the difference between $30,000 in treatment costs and $200,000-plus.

Statins for primary prevention in people with high cholesterol cost approximately $42,000 per QALY at current generic prices. That sounds expensive until you compare it to treating a heart attack ($20,000-$40,000 for the acute event, plus ongoing management) or bypass surgery ($70,000-$200,000).

Hypertension screening and treatment costs approximately $37,100 per life-year saved. Stroke treatment costs $97,000 on average for the acute event alone, not counting long-term disability care and rehabilitation.

Every single preventive intervention is cost-effective by standard healthcare economics measures. Many are actually cost-saving—they save more money than they cost.

So why doesn't the system invest in prevention?

Because the returns are long-term, and American healthcare operates on short-term incentives.

Approximately 21.5% of people with commercial insurance switch insurers every year. Over a two-year period, one in four individuals under age 65 experiences a gap in insurance coverage. The average person doesn't stay with the same insurance company long enough for that company to reap the benefits of prevention.

If an insurance company pays for a diabetes prevention program today, and it successfully prevents diabetes, the savings from not treating diabetes accrue over 20-30 years. The patient, however, will likely have different insurance within 5 years. The company that paid for prevention doesn't get the benefit—their competitor does.

This is called the "wrong pocket problem" in health economics. The investment comes out of one pocket (today's insurer) but the savings go into a different pocket (tomorrow's insurer, or Medicare, or the healthcare system broadly). No individual actor has the incentive to make the investment, even though the investment benefits the system as a whole.

The result: prevention gets deprioritized, underfunded, and ignored. Meanwhile, patients get sick with preventable diseases that cost fortunes to treat.

International Comparisons: Countries That Prioritize Prevention

The United States spent 17.2% of GDP on healthcare in 2024. Other high-income countries averaged 11.2% of GDP, with most spending between 10-12%.

We spend almost double what comparable countries spend, and we get worse results.

U.S. life expectancy in 2016: 78.8 years—the lowest among high-income countries. Life expectancy in other developed nations ranged from 80.7 to 83.9 years.

U.S. infant mortality: 5.8 deaths per 1,000 live births—the highest among comparable countries. Average for other nations: 3.6 per 1,000.

We pay more and die younger. How is this possible?

The spending differential isn't driven by Americans using more healthcare. Utilization rates are largely similar across countries. The difference is price—and how the system is structured.

As mentioned, administrative costs account for 8% of U.S. healthcare spending versus 1-3% in other countries.

Pharmaceutical spending is $1,443 per capita in the U.S. versus $466-$939 in comparable nations.

Physician salaries are substantially higher in the U.S.—generalist physicians (GPs) earn $218,173 here compared to $86,607-$154,126 in other countries.

Despite all this, the real difference is structural: other countries emphasize prevention because their healthcare systems benefit from it.

The United Kingdom's National Health Service spends among the least per capita of comparator countries—substantially less than the U.S. 's $14,775 per person. The NHS emphasizes general practitioners (primary care) as the foundation of the system. GPs focus on prevention, early intervention, and managing chronic conditions before they become severe. Patients register with a GP practice and maintain long-term relationships with their providers.

This longitudinal continuity creates incentive alignment. The NHS pays for prevention today and receives the benefit when disease is prevented tomorrow—because it's the same entity paying for both. There's no "wrong pocket" problem.

Japan's healthcare system requires employers to provide annual health screenings for all employees. The government mandates preventive health checks for people over 40. Screening rates are high, disease is caught early, and the system invests heavily in prevention because it benefits from reduced treatment costs later.

Scandinavian countries similarly emphasize public health, preventive care, and primary care as the foundation of their healthcare systems. They spend less per capita ($7,860 average vs. $14,775) than the U.S. and achieve better health outcomes—not because their medicine is superior, but because their incentive structures reward keeping people healthy rather than treating them when they're sick.

The critical difference: these are single-payer or heavily regulated multi-payer systems where the entity paying for healthcare today is the same entity that benefits from prevention working tomorrow. They have every reason to invest in preventing disease, because they'll save money when disease doesn't occur.

The United States has a fragmented, for-profit system where nobody benefits from long-term prevention because patients churn between insurers every few years. Every actor in the system profits more from disease than from health.

That's not a bug. That is part of the design.

The ACA's Preventive Care Mandate: Small Victory, Limited Impact

The Affordable Care Act required insurance plans to cover certain preventive services without cost-sharing—no copays, no deductibles, just free preventive care. This was a genuine improvement. Over 100 preventive services are now covered, including cancer screenings, immunizations, counseling services, and preventive medications.

An estimated 71 million additional people gained access to preventive services without cost-sharing because of this provision.

Utilization increased for some services. In 2018, screening rates were relatively high for colon cancer (66%), cervical cancer (73%), and breast cancer (72-79%). Routine checkup rates increased 2.7% among the privately insured after the ACA. Flu vaccination rates increased 5.9%.

Yet, many preventive services remain dramatically underutilized.

HPV vaccination: 16.5%.

Zoster (shingles) vaccination: 26.6%.

HIV testing: 45.8%.

The fundamental problem still remained: insurance status is still the dominant factor affecting utilization. The uninsured consistently show lower utilization across virtually all preventive services. Being uninsured matters more than the ACA's free preventive care mandate, because you can't get free preventive care if you don't have insurance.

More importantly, eliminating cost-sharing didn't change the underlying incentive structure. Insurance companies still profit more from disease management than prevention. Providers still get paid more for procedures than for counseling patients about diet and exercise. The healthcare system still generates more revenue when you're sick than when you're healthy.

Making preventive care free was a step forward, but it did not fundamentally realign incentives away from reactive treatment and toward proactive prevention.

Provider Payment Models: Fee-for-Service vs. Value-Based Care

Fee-for-service payment is exactly what it sounds like: providers get paid for each service they deliver. Every office visit, every procedure, every test, every intervention generates a separate payment.

This creates obvious incentive problems. More services equal more revenue. Doing more—whether it's medically necessary or not—gets rewarded. Keeping patients healthy means fewer visits, fewer tests, fewer procedures, less revenue.

The medical literature is clear about the consequences: the U.S. healthcare system devotes the vast majority of expenditures to medical treatment, despite medical treatment accounting for only 10% of premature deaths. Behavioral patterns account for 40% of premature deaths. Genetic predispositions: 30%.

Social circumstances: 15%.

Environmental exposures: 5%.

We spend most of our money on the thing that matters least, and virtually nothing on the things that matter most—because the payment model rewards treatment, not prevention.

Value-based care was supposed to fix this. Instead of paying for volume (number of services), it is supposed to incentivize paying for value (health outcomes achieved). It is supposed to reward providers who keep patients healthy, not providers who do the most procedures.

It hasn't worked.

The overarching goals of value-based payment programs—improving quality and lowering costs—have been largely unmet. The Comprehensive Primary Care Plus (CPC+) model, the largest primary care payment reform effort tested, showed mixed results at best. Multiple inpatient and outpatient value-based purchasing programs have been implemented and evaluated. Their impact has been marginal.

Pay-for-performance programs probably improve some targeted outcomes like childhood immunization rates. Effects on actual patient health outcomes still remain uncertain.

So why hasn't value-based care worked?

First, the incentives are inadequate. Value-based payment programs typically add small bonuses or penalties on top of base fee-for-service payments. The financial incentives aren't large enough to overcome the fundamental structure that rewards doing more.

Second, administrative complexity creates waste. Value-based programs require extensive data collection, reporting, quality measurement, and compliance documentation—creating exactly the kind of administrative burden that drives up costs and burns out providers.

Third, and most fundamentally, value-based care still operates within a for-profit insurance system. As long as insurance companies profit from premium collection and claim denial, as long as pharmaceutical companies profit from high drug prices, as long as hospitals profit from expensive procedures, no amount of tinkering with provider payment models will fix the underlying misalignment of incentives.

You can't count on value-based care to get you out of a system designed to profit on sickness.

Primary Care vs. Specialist Reimbursement

In 2017, specialist physicians earned an average of $399,300. Primary care physicians earned $247,300. The gap: $152,000.

This pay differential tells you everything about what the American healthcare system values. Specialists who do procedures get paid dramatically more than primary care physicians who focus on prevention, chronic disease management, and keeping patients healthy.

Medicare payment data shows the median specialist receives approximately twice the Medicare payments of the median primary care physician. In the second half of 2021, the median primary care physician received $45,962 from Medicare while the median specialist received $85,397—a gap of $39,435.

In 2021, Medicare implemented payment policy changes specifically designed to increase primary care reimbursement and reduce the specialist-primary care gap. The result? The gap decreased by $825. Less than a thousand dollars.

The problem is structural. Medicare operates under budget-neutral requirements—total spending can't increase. If you want to pay primary care physicians more, you have to pay specialists less. Meanwhile, specialist lobbying groups fight viciously against any reduction in their reimbursement.

So the gap persists. Primary care physicians—who could prevent disease, manage chronic conditions, counsel patients on lifestyle changes, catch problems early—earn dramatically less than procedural specialists who treat disease after it's already developed.

Medical students see this pay differential and make rational economic decisions. Why go into primary care and earn $247,000 while dealing with complex patients and time-consuming preventive counseling, when you can specialize and earn $399,000 doing procedures?

The result:

- Primary care physician shortages, especially in underserved areas.
- Longer wait times to see a primary care doctor.
- Less time per appointment.
- Less emphasis on prevention because there's no time and no payment for it.

The system pays specialists to treat disease and underpays primary care physicians who could prevent it. Yet, we wonder why Americans are so sick.

The Human Cost

The reactive model doesn't just waste money. It destroys lives.

David, from our opening example, survived his stroke. But his right hand doesn't work properly anymore. He can't do the skilled work he spent decades learning. He's on disability, living on a fraction of his former income, dealing with chronic pain and limited mobility.

This was preventable. Thirty dollars a month for a statin. A few hundred dollars in annual monitoring. Maybe $2,000 total over two years.

Instead: a stroke, $97,000 in immediate costs, permanent disability, a lifetime of reduced quality of life.

Multiply David's story by millions. People who develop Type 2 diabetes that could have been prevented. Heart attacks that could have been avoided. Cancers caught at Stage 3 that could have been detected at Stage 1. Amputations, dialysis, blindness, strokes—preventable complications of preventable diseases.

We know how to prevent these diseases. The interventions are proven. The cost-effectiveness is documented. Prevention works, and it saves money.

As illustrated in this chapter, the system doesn't profit from prevention. It profits from disease management. So prevention gets ignored, and people get sick with conditions that could have been avoided.

This isn't healthcare. This is a business model that requires human suffering to generate revenue.

Until we build a system that profits from keeping people healthy instead of treating them when they're sick, the suffering will continue.

So now you know that the reactive model isn't broken. It's working exactly as designed—for everyone except the patients.

> *Then, as if it isn't bad enough that the system is incentivized to let us get sick, the part meant to protect us financially will go out of its way to avoid being left with the bill when we do.*

CHAPTER

5 The Preexisting Condition Weapon

This opening scenario is hypothetical, constructed to illustrate a common reality.

Rachel was 28 when she was diagnosed with thyroid cancer. Stage 1, caught early, excellent prognosis. She had surgery to remove her thyroid, followed by radioactive iodine treatment. Six months later, she was cancer-free. Her endocrinologist told her she could expect a normal lifespan with daily thyroid hormone replacement medication.

Two years later, Rachel decided to leave her job at a large corporation to start her own business. She was healthy, energetic, ready to take the risk. All she needed was health insurance.

This was 2012, before the Affordable Care Act's major provisions took effect.

Rachel applied for individual health insurance. She filled out the medical history questionnaire honestly, disclosing her thyroid cancer diagnosis and treatment. She'd been cancer-free for two years. She took one medication daily that cost $20 per month. She saw her endocrinologist twice a year for monitoring. She was, by any reasonable measure, healthy.

The insurance company denied her application.

Not because her prognosis was poor—it was excellent. Not because she required expensive ongoing treatment—she didn't. It was because she had a history of cancer, and that made her a bad risk. The denial letter was brief and final: "We are unable to offer you coverage at this time due to your medical history."

Rachel tried another insurer. Same result. And another. Denied, denied, denied.

She couldn't get health insurance because she'd had cancer. Still, she desperately needed health insurance because she'd had cancer—she needed ongoing monitoring, thyroid medication, regular check-ups to ensure the cancer didn't return.

She had three choices: stay at her corporate job and keep the group insurance that couldn't deny her, pay $1,800 per month for COBRA coverage she couldn't afford as a startup founder, or go without insurance and hope nothing went wrong.

She stayed at the job. The business idea died. Rachel spent the next two years handcuffed to an employer by a cancer diagnosis that no longer affected her health but permanently marked her as uninsurable.

This was legal. This was normal. This was how American healthcare worked until 2014.

What Counted as a Preexisting Condition

Before the Affordable Care Act banned the practice, health insurance companies engaged in "medical underwriting"—where they evaluated applicants' health history to determine whether to offer coverage and at what price.

In theory, this sounds reasonable. Insurance is about risk pooling, and people with expensive medical conditions cost more to cover.

In practice, it was a weapon used to deny coverage to anyone who'd ever been sick.

The list of preexisting conditions that could get you denied was absurdly broad. Chronic conditions, obviously: diabetes, heart disease, asthma, arthritis. Cancer, even if you'd been in remission for years. HIV/AIDS. Hepatitis. Kidney disease. Autoimmune conditions like lupus or rheumatoid arthritis.

Mental health conditions, such as depression, anxiety, bipolar disorder, ADHD, PTSD. If you'd ever been prescribed psychiatric medication or seen a therapist, that went in your file.

Even pregnancy. Yes, pregnancy—a normal biological process—was classified as a preexisting condition in many states. If you were pregnant when applying for insurance, you could be denied. If you'd had pregnancy complications in the past, that could disqualify you for future coverage.

Being a victim of domestic violence was considered a preexisting condition in eight states and the District of Columbia. Insurance companies argued that domestic violence victims had higher healthcare costs due to injuries and mental health treatment, so they charged higher premiums or denied coverage entirely.

Even minor conditions could be used against you. Acne, if you'd been prescribed medication for it. Seasonal allergies. Sleep apnea. High cholesterol, even if well-controlled with cheap generic medication.

The medical underwriting process was invasive and punitive. Insurance companies didn't just ask about your current health—they wanted your complete medical history, often going back years. They requested records from every doctor you'd seen. They scoured your history for anything that might indicate future healthcare costs.

If you made a mistake on your application—forgot to mention that you saw a dermatologist five years ago for a skin rash, or didn't realize that your doctor had noted "possible anxiety" in your chart even though you never followed up—the insurance company could use that as grounds for rescission.

Rescission: The Bait and Switch

Rescission was one of the cruelest practices in pre-ACA health insurance. Here's how it worked:

You apply for insurance. You fill out the medical history questionnaire as honestly and completely as you can remember. The insurance company accepts your application. You start paying premiums every month—$300, $500, $800, whatever the plan costs.

You pay for a year. Two years. Three years. You're a good customer. You rarely use your insurance. Maybe a few doctor visits, some prescriptions, nothing major.

Then you get seriously ill. Cancer. Heart attack. A condition requiring expensive treatment. You file a major claim.

The insurance company then investigates.

They comb through your medical records—all of them, going back years. They're looking for discrepancies between what you reported on your application and what's in your file. Any discrepancy will do.

Did you mention that you saw a chiropractor for back pain six years ago? No? Well, your primary care doctor's notes from seven years ago mention "patient reports occasional back discomfort." You failed to disclose a preexisting condition. Coverage rescinded.

Did you note that your doctor once suggested you might have seasonal allergies, even though you never got tested or treated? No? Preexisting condition not disclosed. Coverage rescinded.

The technicality didn't matter. What mattered was finding any reason—any reason at all—to cancel your coverage retroactively so they wouldn't have to pay your claim.

Rescission didn't just deny you future coverage. It cancelled the coverage you'd already paid for. The insurance company would return your premiums and declare that you had never been insured. Any claims filed during that time? Denied. Any care received? You owed it out of pocket.

People with cancer had their coverage cancelled mid-chemotherapy. People who'd paid premiums for years while healthy got rescinded the moment they actually needed insurance. This was all perfectly legal.

Congressional hearings in the late 2000s exposed the scale of the problem. Insurance company executives were called to testify about their rescission practices. When asked if they would commit to ending rescission except in cases of intentional fraud, they refused.

Because rescission was profitable. Deny coverage to sick people, keep the premiums from when they were healthy, avoid paying expensive claims. From a business perspective, it made perfect sense.

From a human perspective, it was monstrous.

The High-Risk Pool Trap

For people who couldn't get regular insurance due to preexisting conditions, many states offered "high-risk pools"—special insurance programs specifically for people deemed too sick to insure normally.

This sounds like a solution. It wasn't.

First, sixteen states didn't have high-risk pools at all before the ACA. If you lived in one of those states and had a preexisting condition, you had no options in the individual market.

In states that did have high-risk pools, the coverage was prohibitively expensive and inadequate. Premiums were typically 150-200% of standard insurance rates—sometimes more. If regular insurance costs $500 per month, high-risk pool coverage might cost $1,000-$1,500.

Coverage was often capped at levels that were insufficient for serious illness. Annual caps of $50,000 or $75,000 sound like a lot until you're diagnosed with cancer and realize that chemotherapy alone can exceed that in a single year.

Many high-risk pools had waiting periods before coverage actually started—sometimes six months, sometimes a year. If you needed treatment immediately, you were out of luck.

In many states, the pools even had waiting lists. You couldn't just sign up and get coverage—you had to wait for an opening, which might not come for months or years.

The data proves how inadequate high-risk pools were. When the ACA implemented preexisting condition protections in 2014, the biggest coverage gains occurred in states that hadn't had high-risk pools. The sixteen states without pools saw dramatic increases in insurance coverage for people with chronic conditions—proof that the pools, where they existed, weren't actually solving the problem.

High-risk pools were a way to segregate sick people, charge them more, give them less, and pretend the market was working.

The ACA's Victory

On January 1, 2014, the Affordable Care Act's preexisting condition protections took effect.

Suddenly, for the first time in American history, health insurance companies couldn't deny coverage based on medical history.

Guaranteed issue: insurers had to offer coverage to anyone who applied, regardless of health status.

Community rating: insurers could only vary premiums based on age, location, and tobacco use—not on health conditions. Someone with diabetes paid the same premium as someone without it (holding age, location, and smoking status constant).

No annual or lifetime caps: insurers couldn't limit how much they'd pay out over time. If you got cancer and needed expensive treatment, your coverage wouldn't run out.

No rescission except in cases of fraud: insurance companies couldn't cancel your coverage retroactively because you forgot to mention a minor medical issue on your application.

The impact was immediate and substantial.

The Congressional Budget Office estimated the ACA would bring 26 million people onto insurance rolls by 2017. Early expansion allowed 3.1 million young adults to gain coverage by staying on their parents' plans until age 26.

Among adults with chronic conditions specifically, coverage increased by 6-9% depending on the condition and region. People with diabetes saw coverage increase 6.41%. Hypertension: 6.09%. Heart disease: 6.50%. Asthma: 6.37%. People with two or more chronic conditions saw coverage increase 6.39%.

The gains were even larger in some populations. Among community health center patients who were previously uninsured, over 70% of those who gained insurance post-ACA had at least one preexisting condition. Black and Hispanic patients experienced the largest increases, with nearly 19 percentage points more having documented preexisting conditions and access to coverage.

For people with diabetes, the changes were dramatic. Private insurance coverage for Type 1 diabetes showed a 4% decline before the ACA's preexisting condition mandate and an 11% increase after. For people aged 50-59 with Type 1 diabetes, coverage went from -6% before the mandate to +20% after.

The preexisting condition protections didn't just increase coverage—they reduced financial burden. Out-of-pocket spending decreased by $279 for people with preexisting conditions who had non-group insurance. Mental health improved: the policy reduced severe mental distress by 1.44 percentage points among people with preexisting physical health conditions.

People like Rachel—the woman in our opening example—could finally leave their jobs and start businesses without losing access to healthcare. Cancer survivors could get insurance. People with chronic conditions weren't trapped in employer-based coverage or facing bankruptcy from medical bills.

This was genuinely transformative.

Yet, it didn't fix everything. Insurance was still expensive. It was still tied to employment for most people. Insurance companies still denied claims aggressively. The ACA made healthcare accessible for people with preexisting conditions, but it didn't address the underlying profit-driven model that makes American healthcare uniquely terrible.

And the protections remained vulnerable.

The Fragility of Protection

The ACA's preexisting condition protections aren't constitutional rights. They're legislative provisions that can be repealed with a simple majority vote in Congress.

Consequently, from the moment they took effect, powerful interests have been trying to eliminate them.

The 2017 repeal attempts came closest to succeeding. The House passed the American Health Care Act in May 2017, which would have allowed states to waive community rating requirements—effectively letting insurance companies charge people with preexisting conditions higher premiums again.

The Senate tried multiple times to pass repeal legislation. The Better Care Reconciliation Act, the Obamacare Repeal Reconciliation Act, the Graham-Cassidy amendment—all would have gutted preexisting condition protections in various ways.

They failed by the narrowest possible margins. Senator John McCain's famous thumbs-down vote killed the "skinny repeal" attempt. The margin was razor-thin—one vote, after months of intense lobbying and political pressure.

The current administration has made dismantling the ACA a priority. As I write this in January 2026, ACA subsidies that make insurance affordable for millions of Americans are set to expire. The administration is actively pushing to let them lapse, which would make insurance unaffordable even for people who can technically get coverage.

The longest government shutdown in U.S. history happened last November—ultimately about healthcare, about whether to fund ACA subsidies, about whether to maintain the protections that millions of Americans depend on.

Right now, as you read this, people with preexisting conditions are worried about losing access to healthcare. Not someday. Not in some theoretical future. Now.

The threat is compounded by the expansion of "junk" insurance plans that don't have to comply with ACA regulations. Short-term health plans—originally designed to cover brief gaps in coverage—have been expanded to last up to three years. Association health plans allow small businesses to band together and buy coverage that doesn't meet ACA standards.

These plans can exclude preexisting conditions, impose annual and lifetime caps, and charge higher premiums based on health status. They're marketed as "affordable alternatives" to ACA plans, but they're only affordable if you're healthy. If you get sick while covered by a short-term plan, you're on your own.

The expansion of these plans undermines the ACA's protections by siphoning healthy people out of the ACA-compliant insurance pool, leaving sicker people behind and driving up premiums for comprehensive coverage.

State-level attacks continue as well. Some states have requested waivers to modify ACA requirements. Others have refused to enforce consumer protections. The result is a patchwork where your access to coverage depends on which state you live in—exactly the kind of fragmentation that the ACA was supposed to fix.

What's at Stake

Here's what's at risk if preexisting condition protections are eliminated:

Roughly half of non-elderly Americans have some condition that would have been considered a preexisting condition before the ACA. Chronic diseases, past cancer diagnoses, mental health conditions, pregnancy history—conditions that are common, often manageable, but that make you "uninsurable" in a market that allows medical underwriting.

Among people who gained insurance through the ACA, over 70% had at least one preexisting condition. These aren't people looking for a handout. These are people who need access to healthcare to manage chronic conditions, people who would be denied coverage or charged unaffordable premiums without protections.

If the ACA is repealed without a replacement that maintains these protections—and no credible replacement plan has ever been proposed—we go back to pre-2014.

Back to denials.

Back to rescission.

Back to high-risk pools with unaffordable premiums and inadequate coverage.

Back to medical underwriting where having once been sick makes you permanently uninsurable.

Cancer survivors would lose coverage. People with diabetes, heart disease, asthma, mental health conditions—millions of Americans would suddenly be unable to get insurance in the individual market.

This concerns people who are healthy now as well. Eventually, most people develop some chronic condition. Under a system that allows preexisting condition exclusions, getting sick once can mean you're uninsurable for life.

The only people who are never at risk are people who never leave employer-based coverage—which brings us back to job lock, to being trapped by your employer, to the impossibility of starting a business or taking a career risk because you can't afford to lose your health insurance.

The Employer-Insurance Connection

Before the ACA, employer-based insurance partially solved the preexisting condition problem—but only if you never left your job.

The Health Insurance Portability and Accountability Act (HIPAA) of 1996 prohibited group health plans from excluding individuals based on health status. If you had employer-sponsored insurance, the insurer couldn't deny you coverage because you had diabetes or a history of cancer.

However, this protection only applied to group coverage. If you left your job and tried to buy insurance on the individual market, you were back to medical underwriting. Your preexisting conditions could be used to deny you coverage or charge you higher premiums.

So people with chronic conditions were trapped. You couldn't leave your employer-sponsored coverage without losing your only access to insurance. You couldn't start a business. You couldn't take a job at a small company that didn't offer health benefits. You couldn't retire before age 65 when Medicare eligibility kicked in.

Your health history controlled your career choices in ways that had nothing to do with your ability to work or your actual health status.

The ACA broke this trap. For the first time, people with preexisting conditions could leave employer-based coverage and buy insurance in the individual market without being denied or charged prohibitive premiums.

Repealing the ACA would recreate the trap. People with chronic conditions would be handcuffed to their employers again, unable to take career risks, to pursue opportunities, or to retire early—because losing employer-sponsored coverage would mean becoming uninsurable.

Beyond Health Insurance

I know what it's like to be penalized for preexisting conditions—not in health insurance, but in life insurance.

When I applied for life insurance, the company didn't just evaluate my health. They went back to my mother's medical history. She had a heart attack in her 50s. I have no history of heart disease myself. My cholesterol is normal. My blood pressure is fine. I exercise regularly and don't smoke.

My mother's heart attack still meant I was a higher risk. My life insurance premiums were therefore higher than they would have been if my mother hadn't gotten sick decades ago.

This is legal in life insurance. Companies can—and do—discriminate based on family health history, your own health history, genetic test results, anything that suggests you might die sooner and they might have to pay out the policy.

It's worth noting this because it reminds us: the ACA's health insurance protections are an anomaly, not the norm. In every other kind of insurance, companies are allowed to discriminate based on risk factors including health conditions.

Life insurance does it. Disability insurance does it. Long-term care insurance does it.

Health insurance is the only form of insurance where we've decided—temporarily, fragilely—that people shouldn't be penalized for their health history or their family's health history.

Yet, powerful interests want to go back to treating health insurance like any other insurance product: deny the people who need it most, cherry-pick the healthy people who'll pay premiums and never file claims, and thereby maximize profit by minimizing risk.

That's the business model. It's only illegal because of protections that are currently under attack and that could be eliminated at any moment.

The Political Reality

Here's the contradiction at the heart of American healthcare politics: preexisting condition protections are overwhelmingly popular. Polling consistently shows that 70-80% of Americans—including majorities of Republicans—support requiring insurance companies to cover people with preexisting conditions.

Politicians know this. Which is why even politicians who vote to repeal the ACA claim they'll "protect people with preexisting conditions."

It's just that they won't say how, because there is no way to protect people with preexisting conditions without either (a) requiring insurance companies to cover them regardless of health status, which is what the ACA does, or (b) creating a government program that covers everyone, which would be even more dramatic than the ACA.

Every repeal proposal claims it will maintain protections while repealing the law that creates those protections. It's political double-speak designed to obscure the fact that you can't have it both ways.

Insurance companies would love to go back to medical underwriting. Denying expensive patients and cherry-picking healthy ones is enormously profitable. The preexisting condition protections force insurers to cover people who cost money, which cuts into their profits.

The tension is real: popular policy versus industry profits versus political ideology. The result is a constant, grinding threat to protections that millions of people depend on.

Every election cycle, preexisting condition protections are on the ballot. Every congressional session, there are new proposals to undermine them. Every administration has the power to weaken enforcement or expand loopholes.

The protections exist today. They might not exist tomorrow. Millions of Americans live with that uncertainty, knowing that their access to healthcare depends on political battles that have nothing to do with whether they're healthy or sick, whether they need medical care or can afford it.

They depend on whether politicians value human lives more than campaign contributions from the insurance industry.

So far, the protections have survived, but survival isn't the same as security. For people with preexisting conditions—which is to say, for most Americans eventually—security would mean building a healthcare system that doesn't require constant political battles to maintain the basic principle that sick people deserve access to medical care.

We haven't built that system yet. Until we do, the preexisting condition weapon remains loaded, waiting for the next politician willing to pull the trigger.

But if you have insurance, it will protect you, right?

CHAPTER 6

Medical Bankruptcy

The Insured Bankruptcy

This opening scenario is hypothetical, constructed to illustrate a common reality.

Sarah Chen had done everything right. She worked as a high school teacher, carried health insurance through her employer, maintained a modest emergency fund, and paid her bills on time. She owned a small house in the suburbs, drove a reliable used car, and had started saving for her daughter's college education. By any reasonable measure, Sarah was living a responsible, middle-class American life.

Then she found the lump.

The breast cancer diagnosis came on a Tuesday afternoon. Sarah sat in her oncologist's office, her husband gripping her hand, as the doctor outlined the treatment plan: surgery, chemotherapy, radiation. Standard protocol. Good prognosis if they acted quickly. Sarah's insurance was accepted at this hospital system. Everything would be fine.

Sarah believed him about the prognosis. She was less certain about the "fine" part.

Her insurance card listed a $1,800 monthly premium (split with her employer), a $6,000 deductible, and 20% coinsurance after that. The words "out-of-pocket maximum: $14,000" seemed like a lot of money, but manageable if she was careful. She'd saved $8,000 in her emergency fund. They could make it work.

Eighteen months later, Sarah filed for bankruptcy with $127,000 in debt—most of it medical.

This wasn't supposed to happen. She had insurance. She stayed in-network. She got prior authorizations for every procedure. She followed every rule the insurance company set.

But the bills kept coming—and many weren't subject to her out-of-pocket maximum. The $2,400 genetic test her oncologist ordered wasn't covered. The anti-nausea medication that made it possible for her to keep down food required prior authorization that was denied three times before being approved—by which point she'd paid $1,200 out of pocket for doses she couldn't wait for. She hit her $14,000 out-of-pocket maximum in the first three months.

Then the calendar year reset mid-treatment, and she hit it again. $28,000 in out-of-pocket costs over 18 months, just for covered services.

Meanwhile, she'd had to cut back to part-time work, losing $40,000 in income. Her husband took unpaid leave to drive her to appointments when the chemotherapy made it unsafe for her to drive. The medical bills were only part of the story: the lost wages; the credit card debt to cover living expenses while she couldn't work; the retirement savings they'd drained to make ends meet; and the mortgage payments they fell behind on when choosing between the house and her treatment.

By the time she finished treatment, they owed more than they'd ever be able to repay.

Sarah's not unusual. Among non-elderly adults with cancer, more than one-third borrow money or go into debt because of treatment. 3% file for bankruptcy. 46% of patients with commercial insurance reach their maximum out-of-pocket limit in the year of diagnosis. One in two cancer survivors experiences financial toxicity. 25% report material hardship—problems paying medical bills. 34% report psychological hardship—constant worry about medical bills even years after treatment ends.

Sarah had good insurance. She did everything right. It didn't matter.

Then there were the bills she didn't anticipate. The anesthesiologist wasn't in her network, despite the hospital and surgeon being covered. That was an extra $4,200. The pathologist who analyzed her biopsy? Also out of network. Another $1,800. The radiologist who read her mammograms and later her follow-up scans? Out of network for some, in network for others, though Sarah had no way to know which was which when she scheduled the appointments. Each surprise bill arrived weeks or months after the service, long after Sarah thought she knew what she owed.

The insurance company denied coverage for the genetic testing, calling it "not medically necessary," despite her oncologist's insistence that it would guide treatment decisions. Sarah spent hours on hold, filed appeals, eventually paid out of pocket because she needed the results to move forward. The insurance company later approved coverage for a different genetic test—one her doctor said was less comprehensive—but by then Sarah had already paid for the first one.

Her out-of-pocket maximum turned out not to be a maximum at all. It didn't include out-of-network charges. It didn't include the medications her insurance deemed "not on formulary." It reset every January, and her treatment spanned two calendar years. By the time Sarah understood how the math actually worked, she was already $40,000 in debt.

Then she had to stop working. The chemotherapy left her too exhausted to stand in front of a classroom for seven hours a day. She took FMLA leave—unpaid, of course, because her school district's sick leave policy offered two weeks per year and she'd already used that up. Short-term disability paid 60% of her salary, but only after a two-week waiting period, and only for twelve weeks. After that, she went on long-term disability at 50% of her salary, which barely covered the mortgage and car payment, let alone the medical bills still arriving daily in the mail.

Her husband took a second job delivering pizzas on weekends. They stopped saving for their daughter's college fund. They sold Sarah's car—she wasn't driving anyway—and used the money to pay down the credit cards they'd been using to cover the gaps. It wasn't enough. The hospital sent the unpaid balance to collections. The collection agency called twice a day, sometimes more. They threatened to sue. They said they could garnish her husband's wages and place a lien on the house.

Sarah and her husband consulted a bankruptcy attorney on a Friday afternoon, sitting in his fluorescent-lit office while he explained that medical debt was the number one cause of bankruptcy in America: that most people who filed medical bankruptcy had insurance, just like Sarah; that she'd done nothing wrong; that the system was designed this way.

Sarah filed for Chapter 7 bankruptcy three weeks later. She was thirty-nine years old, cancer-free, and financially destroyed. The collections calls stopped. The credit cards were discharged. They kept the house, barely. Sarah's credit score dropped 200 points. She cried when she signed the papers, not from relief but from shame—the deep, humiliating shame of financial failure in a country that equates bankruptcy with moral deficiency.

She'd had insurance. She'd done everything right. It didn't matter.

The Scale of the Crisis

Sarah's story isn't an anomaly. It's the norm.

Medical bankruptcy is the leading cause of personal bankruptcy in the United States. In 2007—the most recent year with comprehensive national data—62.1% of all bankruptcies were medical-related, affecting an estimated 530,000 American families annually. Let that number sink in: more than half a million families every year, financially destroyed by illness. That represents a 50% increase from 2001, when 46.2% of bankruptcies had medical causes. In just six years, the medical bankruptcy rate doubled. The odds that a bankruptcy had a medical cause were 2.4 times higher in 2007 than in 2001.

Here's the statistic that demolishes every comfortable myth Americans tell themselves about health insurance: 75% of people who filed medical bankruptcy had health insurance at the time they got sick.

Read that again. Seventy-five percent. Not the uninsured. Not people who had "failed to plan ahead" or "made bad choices." People who paid their premiums every month. People who carried coverage through their employers or purchased plans on the individual market. People who thought they were protected.

They were wrong.

The assumption that health insurance protects against bankruptcy is one of the most dangerous lies embedded in American healthcare discourse. Insurance provides incomplete, inadequate, and often illusory protection against the financial devastation of serious illness. Having a health insurance card in your wallet means almost nothing when you're diagnosed with cancer, suffer a heart attack, deliver a premature baby, or develop any of the dozens of expensive chronic conditions that plague American adults.

The medical debtors declaring bankruptcy weren't the stereotypical poor and uninsured. They were middle-class homeowners with college educations and stable jobs. Before they got sick, they were teachers and accountants and small-business owners. They were people who'd saved for retirement, paid their taxes, and done everything society told them to do. Then they got sick, and the system bankrupted them anyway.

Medical debt now comprises more than half of all unpaid personal debts sent to collection agencies. One in eight American women carries medical debt. One in eleven men. Nearly one in five households. These aren't statistics about the margins of society—these are numbers that reach deep into the American middle class.

More recent data shows the crisis has only intensified. By 2020, an estimated 17.8% of Americans had medical debt in collections. Among insured adults aged 18-64, one-fifth incurred unaffordable out-of-pocket costs in 2020, and insurance deductibles left another 7% financially vulnerable. Among Medicare beneficiaries—people who theoretically have comprehensive government insurance—out-of-pocket costs averaged $5,460 in 2016. Half of Medicare beneficiaries spent at least 12% of their income on healthcare costs. One-quarter spent at least 23%.

This isn't a healthcare system. It's a bankruptcy-generation machine that happens to sometimes provide medical care as a side effect.

The phrase "medical bankruptcy" itself is a linguistic obscenity unique to the American vocabulary. It shouldn't exist. In no other developed nation do people lose their homes because they got cancer. In no other wealthy country do families choose between chemotherapy and their children's college fund. Medical bankruptcy is as distinctly American as Fourth of July fireworks and just as capable of destroying what it touches.

Increasingly, the people being destroyed are those who thought they were insured. The growth of high-deductible health plans means that "having insurance" has become a technicality rather than a protection. You're covered—until you actually need care. Then you discover that coverage and affordability are entirely separate concepts, and American insurance provides the former while systematically denying the latter.

The underinsured now outnumber the uninsured as victims of medical financial toxicity. These are people who pay premiums every month for plans that offer minimal protection when serious illness strikes. They have insurance cards. They're counted in statistics about coverage rates. Politicians cite these numbers as evidence that the healthcare system is working. But when these people get sick, they go bankrupt at nearly the same rate as the completely uninsured.

Using strict definitions, 27% of non-elderly adults live in families experiencing at least one of three financial strains: high out-of-pocket burdens, medical debt, or financial barriers to needed care. Using broader definitions, that number rises to 45.4%. Nearly half of American adults under 65 face healthcare-related financial distress. This is the water in which we swim, so ubiquitous that we've stopped recognizing it as drowning.

The Affordable Care Act eliminated lifetime caps on coverage and required insurance plans to cover preventive care. These were meaningful reforms, but medical bankruptcy rates haven't significantly decreased since the ACA's passage because the fundamental mechanisms of financial destruction remain intact: high deductibles, narrow networks, surprise billing, and the systematic transfer of financial risk from insurance companies to patients.

The 530,000 families who file for medical bankruptcy each year represent the visible catastrophe. They're the people who've already lost everything. For every family that files bankruptcy, though, there are dozens more teetering on the edge—depleting savings, maxing out credit cards, taking second jobs, borrowing from retirement accounts, asking relatives for money, selling possessions, choosing between medications and rent. Medical debt doesn't just bankrupt people legally. It bankrupts them emotionally, socially, and psychologically long before they ever see a bankruptcy attorney.

This is American healthcare's greatest achievement: making medical bankruptcy so common that it barely registers as news. We've normalized financial destruction by illness. We've made it so ordinary that people like Sarah Chen file bankruptcy, rebuild their credit over seven years, and consider themselves lucky because at least they survived the cancer. The bar for "success" in American healthcare is so low that not dying counts as winning, even if you lose everything else.

How Medical Bankruptcy Happens —Even With Insurance

The mathematics of medical bankruptcy are brutally simple once you understand them. What's complex is the deliberately obscure way these calculations are hidden from patients until after the bills arrive.

Start with a typical employer-sponsored health insurance plan—the kind approximately 160 million Americans rely on. Let's use realistic 2020s numbers: $1,500 per month in premiums (with the employee paying $450 and the employer covering $1,050), an $8,000 annual deductible, and 20% coinsurance after the deductible is met. There's an out-of-pocket maximum listed at $14,000, which sounds reassuringly finite until you read the fine print.

Now suppose you're diagnosed with cancer. Your oncologist recommends surgery followed by chemotherapy and radiation—standard treatment, covered by insurance, nothing experimental. The hospital charges your insurance company $300,000 for your care. This number is largely fictional, pulled from the hospital's chargemaster price list——a master price list containing tens of thousands of charges for every imaginable service, supply, and procedure the hospital might provide—which bears no relationship to the actual cost of providing care, but it's the starting point for all the math that follows.

Your insurance company "negotiates" this down to $200,000 through their contracted rates. You never see this negotiation. It happens in a black box controlled entirely by entities that profit from your confusion.

Here's what you owe:

First, your $8,000 deductible. You pay the first $8,000 of that $200,000 negotiated rate entirely out of pocket. The insurance company pays nothing until you've cleared this hurdle.

After the deductible, you owe 20% coinsurance on the remaining $192,000. That's $38,400.

Your total out-of-pocket cost: $46,400.

But wait—didn't your plan have a $14,000 out-of-pocket maximum?

It did. That maximum, however, doesn't include out-of-network charges. On top of that, your anesthesiologist wasn't in network, even though you had no opportunity to choose your anesthesiologist and you specifically selected an in-network hospital and surgeon. The out-of-network anesthesiologist bills you $4,200, none of which counts toward your out-of-pocket maximum. Neither does the out-of-network pathologist who analyzed your biopsy ($1,800) or the out-of-network radiologist who read your imaging studies ($900).

Add another $6,900 to your total. We're now at $21,900 out of pocket.

That's not all. Your insurance company denies coverage for several medications, tests, and procedures they deem "not medically necessary"—a determination made by insurance company employees who have never examined you and who work for a company whose profit margins improve every time they deny a claim. You appeal. Some denials are overturned. Others aren't. You pay out of pocket for the denied services because you need them to survive, even though your doctor prescribed them and your insurance theoretically covers cancer treatment.

That's another $8,000.

Total so far: $29,900.

Your out-of-pocket maximum resets every January 1st. Your cancer treatment spans two calendar years. You hit your deductible and out-of-pocket maximum twice. Double all the previous numbers—you're now at $59,800.

You can't work during chemotherapy. The chemicals make you too nauseated and exhausted to function. You take FMLA leave, which protects your job but provides zero income. Your employer offers short-term disability that pays 60% of your salary for twelve weeks. After that, long-term disability pays 50% of your salary. Your household income drops by half. The medical bills keep arriving while your paychecks shrink.

Your spouse continues working but now shoulders the full burden of the mortgage, car payments, utilities, groceries, and childcare alone. There's no money left to pay the medical bills. You put them on credit cards. The interest compounds. You start missing mortgage payments. The hospital sends your unpaid balance to collections. The collection agency threatens to sue.

This is how medical bankruptcy happens, even with insurance. Not through a single catastrophic bill but through the accumulation of many large bills arriving while your income has collapsed. The financial damage is like flood water seeping through every crack—impossible to contain once it starts.

The math gets worse if you're unlucky enough to need air ambulance transport ($40,000, usually out of network), if your cancer treatment requires expensive targeted therapies not on your insurance formulary ($15,000 per month), if you develop complications requiring additional surgery, if your insurance company decides halfway through your treatment that you should switch to a different hospital system because they've renegotiated their contracts. Every complication, every unexpected test, every medication adjustment adds thousands to your total.

Here's the cruelest part: none of this is hidden from the insurance companies or hospitals. They know exactly how much you'll owe. They could tell you upfront. They choose not to, because patient confusion is profitable. By the time you understand the financial catastrophe heading your way, you're already thousands of dollars in debt with no realistic way to stop the flood.

The surprise billing crisis exemplifies this perfectly. You choose an in-network hospital. You verify your surgeon is in network. You get prior authorization for the procedure. You do everything right. Then you receive a bill from the anesthesiologist for $8,000 because they don't participate in your insurance network—even though you never chose them, never met them before surgery, and had no opportunity to select an in-network alternative.

This isn't a bug. It's a feature. Anesthesiologists, radiologists, pathologists, and emergency medicine physicians discovered they could make more money by staying out-of-network and balance billing patients for the difference between their charges and what insurance pays. Hospitals tolerate this arrangement because it shifts the financial and reputational burden to individual physicians and away from the hospital system. Insurance companies tolerate it because it keeps premiums lower—they're not covering these out-of-network charges, so they don't need to raise premiums to account for them. Everyone wins except the patient, who receives a bill for thousands of dollars for a service they didn't choose from a provider they didn't select.

Congress passed the No Surprises Act in 2020, which took effect in 2022 and reduced some surprise billing for emergency services and certain ancillary services. But gaps remain. Ground ambulances aren't covered. Many types of out-of-network care still generate surprise bills. In the meantime, the law does nothing about the underlying problem: the systematic transfer of financial risk from insurance companies to patients through high deductibles and coinsurance.

The cases that generate medical bankruptcy aren't usually surprise bills, though those don't help. The real damage comes from predictable, unavoidable costs that insurance simply doesn't cover adequately. When your cancer treatment costs $300,000 and your insurance makes you pay $50,000 of it, that's not a surprise. That's the system working exactly as designed. The insurance company collected premiums from you for years while you were healthy. Now that you're sick and need the coverage you paid for, they've structured the benefits to ensure you'll pay tens of thousands out of pocket while they continue profiting.

This is the dark genius of modern American health insurance: socializing the revenue collection through premiums while privatizing the financial risk through deductibles and coinsurance. Everyone pays in. Only the sick pay out. When the sick can't pay, they go bankrupt, their debts are discharged or settled for pennies on the dollar, and the system continues extracting premiums from the next cohort of healthy people who believe their insurance cards will protect them.

It won't. Not when it matters. Not when you're sick. That's when you'll learn that "having insurance" and "being protected from bankruptcy" are two entirely different things.

The Uninsured vs. The Underinsured

If you're completely uninsured in America and you need emergency surgery, the hospital bills you the full chargemaster price. No negotiation. No contracted rate. The highest possible number the hospital can generate. A three-day hospital stay can easily reach $100,000. A premature baby requiring NICU care can generate $500,000 in bills. A serious car accident with multiple surgeries can top $1 million.

These numbers are bankrupting. They're also increasingly irrelevant to understanding the medical bankruptcy crisis, because the uninsured are no longer the primary victims. That distinction now belongs to the underinsured—people who have coverage that's technically insurance but functionally inadequate when serious illness strikes.

The growth of high-deductible health plans has fundamentally changed who files medical bankruptcy. These plans require patients to pay thousands out of pocket before insurance covers anything beyond preventive care. Bronze marketplace plans—the cheapest option on the ACA exchanges—commonly have deductibles exceeding $7,500 for individuals. Many employer-sponsored plans now feature deductibles of $5,000 or more. Even gold-level marketplace plans can require $2,000-$3,000 in deductible spending before insurance starts paying.

For healthy people, high-deductible plans make financial sense.

The premiums are lower. You're gambling that you won't get sick, and most years you win that gamble. But when you lose—when you develop cancer or suffer a heart attack or deliver a baby with complications—you lose catastrophically. The deductible that seemed manageable in theory becomes insurmountable when paired with coinsurance, out-of-network charges, denied claims, and lost income from being too sick to work.

The underinsured face a particularly cruel version of medical bankruptcy because they're doing everything they're supposed to do. They're paying premiums. They're insured. They believed the American promise that health insurance protects against financial catastrophe. Then they get sick and discover that their insurance pays for almost nothing until they've spent thousands out of pocket—money they don't have and can't borrow.

The gap between what insurance covers and what healthcare costs has widened into a chasm. Employers have steadily shifted more costs to employees through higher deductibles, larger coinsurance percentages, narrower networks, and formularies that exclude expensive medications. This cost-shifting is marketed as giving patients "more skin in the game" and encouraging them to be "wise healthcare consumers." In reality, it means that middle-class families with employer-sponsored insurance go bankrupt at rates approaching those of the uninsured.

Consider the arithmetic: if you earn $60,000 per year and face an $8,000 deductible plus 20% coinsurance on a $100,000 hospitalization, you owe $26,400 out of pocket. That's 44% of your annual gross income. After taxes, rent, food, utilities, and other non-negotiable expenses, that $26,400 is impossible to pay. You're employed. You're insured. You're bankrupt.

The truly uninsured face a different set of horrors. They avoid care entirely until conditions become life-threatening. They show up to emergency rooms with late-stage cancers that could have been treated if caught earlier. They leave hospitals against medical advice because they know they can't pay. They're quoted chargemaster prices—the highest possible charges—because they lack insurance companies to negotiate rates down. They're charged $15 for an aspirin, $50 for a box of tissues, $100 for a nurse to hand them a pill they could have taken at home for pennies.

Increasingly, though, the uninsured and underinsured face similar outcomes: medical debt they cannot pay, collections calls they cannot stop, and eventual bankruptcy they cannot avoid. The difference is that the underinsured believed they were protected. They paid premiums every month for that protection. They sacrificed other spending to afford health insurance because they were taught that coverage would safeguard their families. Then they got sick and learned that their insurance was largely decorative—present on paper, useless in practice.

The medical debt statistics reflect this reality. Among non-elderly adults, 27% live in families experiencing high out-of-pocket burdens, medical debt, or financial barriers to care using strict definitions. That percentage rises to 45.4% using broader definitions. These aren't primarily the uninsured. These are people with coverage inadequate to protect them from financial distress when they need healthcare.

Medicare beneficiaries—elderly Americans with government insurance—face the same problem. Medicare covers many services but requires substantial cost-sharing. Supplemental insurance helps but doesn't eliminate out-of-pocket costs. The average Medicare beneficiary spent $5,460 out of pocket in 2016. Half spent at least 12% of their income on healthcare. One-quarter spent at least 23%. And Medicare is generally more generous than private insurance. The non-elderly face even higher relative burdens.

The shift from uninsured to underinsured as the primary bankruptcy population reveals something important about American healthcare's evolution. We've successfully reduced the uninsured rate through the ACA. Coverage has expanded. At the same time, we've simultaneously reduced the value of that coverage through higher cost-sharing. We're insuring more people while protecting them less. It's a shell game where the coverage percentages look good in press releases while the medical bankruptcy rate barely budges because the coverage isn't adequate.

This bait-and-switch allows politicians and insurance executives to claim success—look at all the people with insurance!—while ignoring that the insurance they have is increasingly worthless when they're actually sick. We've made coverage mandatory while making it simultaneously inadequate. We've forced people to buy a product that doesn't deliver the protection it claims to provide.

The woman who yelled at me over the phone—the mother with employer-provided insurance who refused to take her son with new neurological symptoms to the emergency room because she was terrified of the cost—had insurance. She was paying premiums every month. Yet, those premiums bought her nothing except fear: fear that using her coverage would bankrupt her family; that seeking necessary care would generate bills she couldn't pay; that doing the right thing medically would be the wrong thing financially.

That fear is rational. She understood, probably from experience, that "having insurance" wouldn't protect her from a $10,000 ER bill after deductibles and coinsurance. She understood that her insurance company would fight to deny coverage. She understood that even if the visit was eventually covered, she'd be fighting with billing departments and insurance companies for months while collection agencies called and her credit score tanked. So she chose to risk her son's health rather than risk her family's financial survival.

That's not a healthcare system. That's a protection racket that charges premiums for coverage that evaporates when you actually need it. That racket doesn't distinguish between the uninsured and underinsured when it comes to medical bankruptcy. It bankrupts both, just through slightly different mechanisms.

Medical Debt Collection Practices

The bills start arriving two to three weeks after your hospital discharge. They come from different providers: the hospital, the surgeon, the anesthesiologist, the radiologist, the lab that processed your blood work, the medical supply company that provided equipment, the ambulance company, the emergency physician, the pathologist. Each bills separately. Each has a different timeline. Each uses slightly different formatting that makes comparing charges nearly impossible.

You call the hospital billing department to set up a payment plan. They offer you twenty-four months to pay off a $40,000 balance. That's $1,667 per month—more than your mortgage payment. You explain that's impossible. They offer forty-eight months. That's still $833 per month. You explain that you're on disability leave at 60% of your normal salary and your spouse is working extra hours just to cover basic living expenses. The billing representative tells you there's nothing more they can do. They suggest you apply for financial assistance—a program you've never heard of and which they don't explain. You ask for details. They transfer you to a customer support line that eventually disconnects.

You miss the first payment deadline because you literally don't have the money. A second notice arrives. You call again, speak to a different representative, negotiate a smaller monthly payment of $250 that you still can't really afford but agree to anyway. You make two payments. The third month, your car needs $800 in repairs and you have to choose between fixing the car your spouse needs to get to work and paying the hospital bill. You choose the car. You plan to catch up next month.

You don't catch up. Instead, you receive a letter from a collection agency. The hospital has sold your debt. The collection agency owns it now, having likely paid pennies on the dollar for the right to pursue you for the full amount plus fees and interest. The letters from the collection agency are more aggressive than the hospital's. They threaten legal action. They call daily, sometimes multiple times. They call your workplace. They threaten to garnish your wages, to place a lien on your house, to destroy your credit rating if you don't pay immediately.

You explain that you can't pay immediately. You offer the same $250 per month you'd arranged with the hospital. The collection agency wants $1,000 per month minimum. You explain that's impossible. They say they'll see you in court.

They're not bluffing. In Virginia alone, 36% of hospitals collectively filed 20,054 lawsuits and 9,232 wage garnishment cases over medical debt in a single study period. These hospitals pursued patients for inflated medical charges in court and garnished paychecks from low-income residents—people who often qualified for financial assistance programs the hospitals never told them existed.

The pattern repeats across the country. Hospitals sue patients, win judgments by default because many defendants don't appear in court (they're working, they're sick, they can't afford attorneys, they don't understand the legal system), and then garnish wages directly from paychecks. Some hospitals garnish wages while patients are still receiving ongoing treatment at those same hospitals. The hospital provides your chemotherapy on Tuesday and garnishes your paycheck on Friday.

The lawsuits don't distinguish between for-profit and nonprofit hospitals. Nonprofit hospitals—institutions that receive tax exemptions because they're supposed to provide community benefit—sue patients for medical debt at similar rates to for-profit hospitals. These nonprofit hospitals are required by law to provide charity care to qualifying patients. Yet they routinely sue patients who would have qualified for that charity care if anyone had bothered to inform them the programs existed.

The math is obscene. Many nonprofit hospital systems maintain billion-dollar endowments while simultaneously pursuing six-figure lawsuits against patients earning poverty-level wages. Hospital CEO compensation at major nonprofit systems regularly exceeds $1 million annually—sometimes reaching $10 million or more—while the institutions they lead garnish the wages of single mothers working as nursing assistants for $14 per hour.

When journalists and researchers exposed these practices in Virginia hospitals, publishing details of the lawsuits and wage garnishments, the hospitals responded to the bad publicity by measurably decreasing their legal filings. This proves the hospitals understood their behavior was indefensible. They weren't pursuing necessary collections to remain solvent. They were engaging in aggressive collections because it was profitable and because no one was watching. When someone started watching, they pulled back—not because the debt disappeared or the patients suddenly became able to pay, but because the reputational damage exceeded the financial gain.

The credit score destruction compounds the damage. Medical debt in collections remains on credit reports for years. The reporting timeframe has been shortened by recent policy changes, but the impact while present is severe. A medical collections entry drops your credit score by 100 points or more. That lower score makes it harder to rent apartments, secure car loans, get approved for mortgages, and sometimes even pass background checks for employment.

Medical debt doesn't just bankrupt you in the narrow legal sense—it exiles you from the economic mainstream.

You can't move to a better apartment. You can't finance reliable transportation. You can't buy a home. You can't access credit for emergencies. The financial toxicity of medical debt spreads through every aspect of your economic life, limiting your options and trapping you in poverty long after the original illness has resolved.

The cascading effects reach beyond pure economics into social determinants of health. Among insured Americans with difficulty paying medical bills, 34% were unable to pay for food, heat, or housing. These aren't separate problems—they're the same problem manifesting across domains. Medical debt leaves people unable to pay utility bills, unable to keep homes adequately heated or cooled, unable to afford sufficient food. It worsens food insecurity and housing instability, which are themselves powerful predictors of adverse health outcomes.

The cruelty here is almost fractal—you can examine it at any scale and find the same pattern of suffering. A patient gets sick, accumulates medical debt, can't pay, gets sued, has wages garnished, can't afford rent, becomes homeless, gets sicker from lack of housing, accumulates more medical debt. The system generates its own demand in a vicious cycle of disease, debt, and desperation.

15% of insured Americans with medical bill difficulties took out high-interest payday loans—predatory financial products that trap borrowers in debt spirals. 42% took on extra jobs or worked additional hours, further damaging their health through stress and exhaustion while sick or recovering. These aren't choices. These are desperation moves by people watching their lives disintegrate under the weight of medical bills they cannot pay for services they had no choice but to receive.

The collection agencies know this. The hospitals know this. They pursue collections anyway because the system incentivizes them to do so. Hospitals can write off unpaid debt as charity care for tax purposes while simultaneously pursuing aggressive collections. They can claim they're providing community benefit while suing community members. They can present themselves as healing institutions while actively destroying the financial health of the patients they claim to serve.

Meanwhile, the patients have no recourse. You can't refuse treatment for life-threatening illness. You can't negotiate prices in advance—hospitals won't tell you what services will cost. You can't shop around for better deals while bleeding out in an emergency room. You're trapped in a system that generates debt you cannot avoid and then punishes you viciously for failing to pay bills you never agreed to in amounts you never knew until after services were rendered.

The medical debt collection industry exists only because American healthcare is structured to generate unpayable bills. In countries with universal healthcare, there's no medical debt collection industry because there's no medical debt. The industry's entire existence is testament to healthcare system failure, and its practices—suing sick people, garnishing poverty wages, destroying credit, driving families into homelessness—are testaments to moral bankruptcy far more profound than the financial bankruptcy inflicted on patients.

The Hospitals' Role

Every hospital in America maintains a document called a "chargemaster"—a master price list for everything the hospital might provide. These prices are completely arbitrary, bearing no relationship to the actual cost of providing care or to prices charged by competing hospitals. A single dose of acetaminophen might be listed at $15. A bag of saline solution might cost $800. The same MRI that costs $400 at an independent imaging center might be billed at $4,000 by the hospital.

The chargemaster serves multiple purposes, none of them beneficial to patients. Insurance companies negotiate discounts off these inflated prices, which makes the discounts appear generous even when the final negotiated rate is still far above cost. Uninsured patients get charged the full chargemaster rate—the highest possible price—because they lack negotiating power. This overall price inflation creates a system where everyone involved can claim they're offering discounts while still generating massive profits.

The complete arbitrariness of chargemaster pricing is evident when you compare prices across hospitals. Hospitals in the same city, providing essentially identical services, charge vastly different amounts. Not 10% different. Not 20% different. Different by factors of three, five, sometimes ten. These price variations don't reflect differences in quality or outcomes. They reflect the lack of any rational pricing mechanism in American healthcare. Hospitals charge whatever they think they can get away with, adjusting prices based on what their competitors charge, what insurance companies will pay, and how aggressive they want to be in pursuing uninsured patients.

Federal price transparency rules, implemented in 2021, require hospitals to publish their chargemaster prices and negotiated rates with insurance companies. Compliance has been poor. Many hospitals have made their price lists technically available while ensuring they're nearly impossible to find or interpret. Others have published files so large and complex that meaningful comparison is impossible without specialized software. The hospitals that have genuinely complied have often seen their prices undercut by competitors, punishing transparency while rewarding continued opacity.

Even when prices are published, they're almost useless for patients trying to estimate costs. You don't know in advance which services you'll need. You don't know which specific physicians will be involved in your care. You don't know if complications will arise requiring additional procedures, and you certainly don't know which services will be denied by insurance, leaving you responsible for the full charge. Price transparency is theoretical. Price unpredictability is the lived reality.

Financial assistance programs add another layer of dysfunction.

The Affordable Care Act requires nonprofit hospitals to maintain financial assistance policies and to make reasonable efforts to determine patient eligibility before pursuing collections. Many nonprofit hospitals theoretically offer charity care that would eliminate or reduce bills for low-income patients. In practice, these programs are systematically underutilized because hospitals don't advertise them, don't screen patients for eligibility, and don't inform patients that help exists until after aggressive collections have already begun—if they inform them at all.

Patients who qualify for charity care often end up in collections and sometimes in court because no one told them to apply for assistance. Hospitals claim they make the programs available. However, "available" and "accessible" are very different things. Burying information about financial assistance in small print on page fifteen of a thirty-page admission packet while the patient is sedated for emergency surgery is not genuine availability. Not training front-line billing staff to screen for eligibility is not genuine availability. Requiring extensive documentation that low-income patients struggle to gather is not genuine availability.

The research on Virginia hospitals found that hospitals sued patients who would have qualified for charity care. They garnished wages from people earning poverty-level incomes who should have had their bills reduced or eliminated entirely. This wasn't accidental. It was systematic institutional failure—or, more accurately, systematic institutional success at extracting maximum revenue regardless of patient ability to pay or legal obligations to provide charity care.

The nonprofit hospital designation itself deserves scrutiny. Nonprofit hospitals receive significant tax advantages—federal and state income tax exemptions, property tax exemptions, and exemption from sales taxes. These tax benefits are justified by the purported community benefit hospitals provide, including charity care for indigent patients. Yet, many nonprofit hospital systems provide charity care at levels far below the value of their tax exemptions. They accumulate enormous reserves and endowments while providing minimal benefit to their communities.

Executive compensation at nonprofit hospitals further exposes the fiction of "nonprofit" status. CEOs of major nonprofit hospital systems routinely earn $1 million to $10 million or more annually. These aren't salaries at struggling community hospitals—they're compensation packages at wealthy institutions with billion-dollar operating budgets and massive endowments. The "nonprofit" designation has become a tax shelter rather than a genuine indicator of community-oriented healthcare delivery.

Meanwhile, these wealthy nonprofit hospitals sue patients for medical debt, garnish wages, place liens on homes, and send patients to collections at rates comparable to for-profit hospitals. The tax-exempt status doesn't translate into patient-protective policies. It translates into accumulated institutional wealth while individual patients face financial ruin.

For-profit hospitals are even more aggressive. They openly prioritize shareholder returns and explicitly optimize for revenue extraction. They're more likely to sue patients, more likely to charge maximum prices, more likely to locate facilities in wealthy areas while avoiding uninsured populations, and more likely to cut services that don't generate profit. In practice, the difference between for-profit and nonprofit hospital collections is often minimal. Both will bankrupt you. The for-profit hospital is just more honest about its priorities.

The hospital industry collectively maintains that aggressive collections are necessary for financial viability. This is largely false. Uncompensated care—care provided without payment—represents a small fraction of hospital operating budgets, typically 2-6%. Hospitals build this uncompensated care into their pricing models. They charge everyone more to cover the costs of those who can't pay. The system is already designed to socialize those losses across all patients and insurers. The aggressive collections aren't about institutional survival. They're about maximizing revenue and minimizing uncompensated care percentages that might affect credit ratings or investor confidence.

The contradiction is stark: hospitals claim they must pursue aggressive collections to remain financially stable, while simultaneously accumulating reserves, building new facilities, expanding into additional markets, and paying executives millions. If collections were truly about survival, we'd see hospitals on the brink of closure. Instead, we see hospital systems building billion-dollar empires while suing patients earning minimum wage.

As I've already pointed out, this isn't healthcare. It is at its core a wealth extraction scheme that happens to provide medical services as a byproduct. The hospitals' primary function in this scheme is to generate maximal bills from maximal prices and to pursue those bills as aggressively as possible without triggering enough public outrage to prompt regulatory intervention. They succeed at this function brilliantly. Patients go bankrupt. Hospitals thrive. The system works exactly as designed—just not for the people it claims to serve.

Why This Only Happens in America

Medical bankruptcy doesn't exist in Canada. Nor in the United Kingdom. Or France, Germany, Japan, Australia, South Korea, or any other developed nation with a functional healthcare system. This isn't because people in those countries don't get sick. Cancer exists everywhere. Heart disease exists everywhere. Diabetes, kidney failure, premature births, and traumatic injuries all occur at similar rates across developed nations. What doesn't occur everywhere is financial annihilation from medical bills.

The reason is simple: other countries have healthcare systems designed to provide healthcare, not to generate profit. They have universal coverage systems that pool risk across entire populations, cap out-of-pocket costs at truly manageable levels, and separate healthcare financing from individual financial catastrophe.

In the United Kingdom, the National Health Service provides care free at point of service. If you develop cancer, you receive treatment. There's no bill. No deductible. No coinsurance. No surprise charges from out-of-network anesthesiologists. You don't navigate insurance company denials or fight about whether a test was "medically necessary." You're sick, you need care, you receive care. The end. The NHS is funded through general taxation, which means healthcare costs are progressive—wealthy people pay more, sick people aren't bankrupted. This is what actual health insurance looks like.

Canada operates a similar model. Provincial health insurance covers necessary medical services without direct charges to patients. If you have a heart attack in Toronto, you're treated at a hospital, and you leave without a bill. You might pay small amounts for prescription drugs or for upgraded hospital rooms, but catastrophic medical expenses don't exist. There's no medical debt because there are no medical bills to put you in medical bankruptcy. The concept doesn't translate.

Germany requires all residents to carry health insurance, either through statutory health insurance (covering ~90% of the population) or private insurance. German insurance, however, is nothing like American insurance. Statutory plans have strict cost-sharing limits. Out-of-pocket costs are capped at 2% of gross income, and just 1% for those with chronic conditions. Two percent of income. Not two percent before hitting your deductible—two percent total, forever, maximum. A German family earning €50,000 annually pays a maximum of €1,000 out of pocket per year for all healthcare costs (roughly $1,100 of $58,000). There's no mechanism for medical bankruptcy when out-of-pocket costs are systematically limited to amounts working families can pay.

France combines public insurance with supplemental private coverage. The public system covers a large percentage of costs, and supplemental insurance covers most of the rest. Typical out-of-pocket costs are minimal. Cancer treatment doesn't bankrupt French families because the insurance actually insures it. It covers what it claims to cover. Co-pays and deductibles exist but are tiny compared to American cost-sharing. The entire system is designed around the principle that sick people shouldn't also be financially destroyed.

Japan requires universal coverage and regulates prices strictly. The government sets prices for all medical services and drugs. Hospitals can't charge arbitrary amounts because prices are standardized nationally. Patients pay 30% coinsurance, but total out-of-pocket costs are capped at levels based on income. High-income families pay maximum monthly out-of-pocket costs around ¥250,000 (roughly $1,700). Lower-income families pay far less. Expensive treatments like cancer care automatically trigger these caps, protecting families from catastrophic expenses. Medical bankruptcy is essentially unknown because the system doesn't generate unpayable bills.

Australia's Medicare system covers hospital care and physician visits. Private insurance exists but supplements the public system rather than replacing it. Out-of-pocket costs exist but are capped and relatively low. Pharmaceutical costs are subsidized through the Pharmaceutical Benefits Scheme, which limits what patients pay for medications regardless of the drug's actual cost. The system ensures that serious illness causes medical problems, not financial ones.

The consistent pattern across all these countries is that healthcare costs are collectivized and capped. Nobody faces unlimited liability for medical expenses. Nobody goes bankrupt because they got cancer. These societies have decided that healthcare risk should be spread across entire populations rather than concentrated on sick individuals and their families. It's not complicated policy—it's basic moral decency codified into healthcare financing structures.

The United States is the outlier. We're the only developed nation that allows—and actively facilitates—medical bankruptcy. We treat healthcare as a consumer product rather than a human necessity. We allow hospitals to charge arbitrary prices, insurance companies to deny coverage for necessary care, and collection agencies to sue sick people for debts they cannot pay. We've built a system that generates medical bankruptcy as its natural output, and we've decided this is acceptable.

American politicians and healthcare industry executives claim that universal healthcare would be too expensive, that it would reduce quality, and create waiting lists and rationing. These are lies. Every other developed nation spends far less per capita on healthcare than the United States while achieving better health outcomes and universal coverage. The U.S. spent 17.2% of GDP on healthcare in 2024, more than 50% higher than comparable countries (which average 11.2%) —while leaving millions uninsured or underinsured and generating the developed world's only medical bankruptcy crisis.

The waiting list argument is particularly dishonest. America has waiting lists too—they're just called "I can't afford that procedure so I'll wait and hope the problem resolves itself" or "I'm waiting until next year when my deductible resets" or "I'm waiting to see if the insurance company approves coverage." We ration care through price rather than through queues, which means poor people wait forever while rich people access care immediately. Other countries ration by need, treating urgent cases quickly and making less urgent cases wait. This is obviously more equitable, but equity isn't the American healthcare system's goal. Profit is.

The quality argument is similarly false. American healthcare quality is inconsistent and often poor compared to other developed nations. We rank poorly on infant mortality, maternal mortality, life expectancy, and management of chronic diseases. Our best hospitals are world-class, but our average outcomes are mediocre and our worst outcomes are catastrophic. Meanwhile, countries with universal coverage consistently rank higher on overall health metrics. The healthcare Americans receive isn't superior. It's just more expensive and more likely to bankrupt us.

What's true is that universal healthcare would be expensive for the government. It would require substantial tax increases, particularly on high earners. That said, those tax increases would replace the premiums, deductibles, and coinsurance Americans currently pay. For most families, the math favors higher taxes and eliminates medical bills. You'd pay more in taxes and less to insurance companies, and you'd have actual coverage that actually protected you from bankruptcy when sick.

The American healthcare industry opposes this because it would reduce their profits. Insurance companies would lose their massive administrative overhead and profit margins. Hospitals would lose their ability to charge arbitrary prices. Pharmaceutical companies would face negotiated pricing. The entire industry would shrink from its current bloated state to something more resembling healthcare systems in other countries—smaller, more efficient, less profitable, and vastly more effective at actually providing healthcare to populations.

Medical bankruptcy exists in America because we've chosen to preserve healthcare industry profits over protecting citizens from financial catastrophe. It's not an accident. It's not an unavoidable consequence of providing high-quality care. It's a policy choice, made repeatedly, to prioritize corporate profits over human welfare. Other countries made different choices. They don't have medical bankruptcy. We could make the same choice. We haven't.

The cruelty is the point, or at least it's an acceptable side effect. A system that bankrupts 530,000 families annually for the crime of getting sick is a system that values money over life, profit over people, and corporate interests over human dignity. We could change this tomorrow if we wanted to. We just don't want it badly enough to overcome industry lobbying and political resistance. So the bankruptcies continue, year after year, while we pretend this is normal and unavoidable. It’s simply the price of freedom, quality, innovation or whatever lie we're currently telling ourselves to justify the unjustifiable.

The Psychological and Social Cost

The bankruptcy attorney's office was fluorescent-lit and institutional, filled with particleboard furniture and motivational posters about "fresh starts" and "new beginnings." Sarah sat across from a lawyer who'd clearly delivered this speech hundreds of times, his tone somewhere between sympathetic and bored as he explained that her medical debt could be discharged through Chapter 7 bankruptcy. Her credit score would tank. She'd struggle to get approved for loans or rental applications for seven years. At least the collection calls would stop. The lawsuits would cease. The debt would be gone.

Sarah signed the papers through tears. Not tears of relief—tears of shame so profound they made her physically sick. She'd done everything right: worked hard, paid her bills, saved money, carried insurance. She'd gotten cancer through no fault of her own, followed her doctors' recommendations exactly, and still ended up here, in a bankruptcy attorney's office, admitting financial failure. The shame was crushing, not because bankruptcy represented actual moral failure, but because America treats financial collapse as a character flaw rather than a systemic outcome.

The psychological damage of medical bankruptcy extends far beyond credit scores and legal paperwork. It's the corrosive shame of being unable to pay for your own healthcare in a society that equates financial success with moral worth. It's the humiliation of collection calls at work, where coworkers overhear someone demanding money you don't have for medical bills you didn't choose. It's the degradation of explaining to your children why you're selling their belongings, why you can't afford their school field trips anymore, why everything changed after Mommy got sick.

Medical bankruptcy doesn't just destroy finances. It destroys relationships. Marriages collapse under the stress of unpayable medical debt. Couples fight about money constantly—whose fault it is, what they should have done differently, whether they should sell the house, whether bankruptcy is the right choice. The financial trauma compounds the medical trauma. You're recovering from cancer while watching your marriage disintegrate. You survived the illness but your relationship didn't survive the bills.

The statistics bear this out: medical debt is cited as a contributing factor in significant percentages of divorces, though exact numbers are difficult to isolate because couples rarely cite a single cause. What's clear is that financial stress destroys relationships, and medical debt creates uniquely intense financial stress because it's unexpected, often massive, and feels profoundly unjust. You got sick. You needed care. Why is your family being punished for that?

Parents feel the guilt acutely. They watch their children's opportunities narrow because medical bills consumed the college fund, the house down payment, the security that middle-class parents are supposed to provide. They explain why there's no money for sports equipment, music lessons, or the class trip to Washington, D.C. They explain that Mommy or Daddy needed expensive treatment and now we're poor. They watch their children internalize the lesson that medical care costs more than anything else their family values—more than education, recreation, and saving for the future. This is the lesson American healthcare teaches children: if you get sick, you'll lose everything.

Elderly patients lose retirement savings accumulated over decades. A lifetime of careful planning, decades of saving and investing, wiped out by three months in a nursing home or a year of cancer treatment. Patients in their seventies and eighties file bankruptcy, destroying credit they'll never have time to rebuild, losing homes they'll never be able to buy again. They spend their final years in poverty after spending their prime years working and saving for a security that evaporated the moment they got sick.

The trauma is compounded by the capriciousness. You didn't choose to get sick. You didn't choose your insurance plan's inadequate coverage—your employer chose it, or it was the only plan you could afford on the marketplace. You didn't choose the hospital's prices—they were set arbitrarily without your input. You didn't choose to have an out-of-network anesthesiologist—they were assigned without your knowledge. None of the decisions that led to your bankruptcy were decisions you actually made, yet you bear all the consequences.

This creates a particular flavor of trauma: the trauma of unchosen outcomes. It's one thing to make risky financial decisions and suffer the consequences. It's entirely different to follow all the rules, make reasonable choices, and still end up bankrupt because the system is designed to bankrupt you. The helplessness breeds depression and anxiety. You learn that doing everything right doesn't protect you, that planning carefully doesn't matter, that being responsible means nothing when the healthcare system decides to financially destroy you.

Some people develop PTSD from the financial trauma of medical debt. Not metaphorical trauma—actual, diagnosable post-traumatic stress disorder. They experience intrusive thoughts about medical bills. They have panic attacks when mail arrives or when the phone rings. They avoid opening mail for weeks because they can't face more bills. They startle at sounds that remind them of collection calls. The financial trauma sits alongside and compounds the medical trauma, creating a layered psychological disaster that requires its own treatment—treatment they often can't afford because they're bankrupted by the original medical bills.

The choice between treatment and financial survival creates its own psychological hell. Cancer patients skip chemotherapy doses to avoid accumulating more debt. Diabetics ration insulin to make prescriptions last longer. Heart disease patients avoid cardiac rehabilitation because they can't afford the co-pays. They know they're compromising their health. They know they're reducing their chances of survival or recovery. They choose financial preservation over medical optimization because American healthcare forces them to make that choice.

This is torture. Not metaphorical torture—actual torture. Creating situations where people must choose between health and financial survival, knowing that either choice leads to suffering, is torture by any reasonable definition. We're torturing sick people for being sick. We're punishing cancer patients for having cancer. We're bankrupting heart attack survivors for surviving, and we're doing it systematically, at scale, to hundreds of thousands of families every year.

The social costs radiate outward in circles. Medical bankruptcy affects not just the person who was sick but their entire family, their children's opportunities, their parents' support systems. It affects communities—neighborhoods where multiple families are struggling with medical debt simultaneously, where everyone knows someone who's been bankrupted by healthcare costs. It affects trust in institutions—why follow rules if following rules doesn't protect you? Why believe in the American Dream if doing everything right still leads to bankruptcy?

The shame extends into social isolation. People don't talk about medical bankruptcy. It's too humiliating, too stigmatized. So people suffer alone, convinced they're the only ones who couldn't handle medical bills, the only ones who failed to plan adequately, the only ones weak enough to let illness destroy them financially. They don't realize that 529,999 other families file medical bankruptcy every year. They don't realize this is normal, expected, designed into the system. They think it's their personal failure rather than systemic failure.

This isolation prevents collective action. If people realized how common medical bankruptcy is, how many of their neighbors and coworkers and friends are one illness away from financial catastrophe, maybe they'd demand systemic change. But the shame keeps people quiet. The stigma prevents organization. So the bankruptcies continue, each family convinced they're alone in their failure, each person carrying shame they don't deserve for outcomes they couldn't control.

The cruelty of medical bankruptcy isn't just economic—it's psychological, social, and moral. It's the cruelty of punishing people for biology; destroying families for seeking healthcare; making children pay for their parents' illnesses. It's the cruelty of teaching people that no amount of planning or responsibility will protect them if they get sick. It's the cruelty of a society that could easily prevent this suffering but chooses not to because doing so would reduce corporate profits.

Medical bankruptcy inflicts trauma on top of trauma, shame on top of suffering, and isolation on top of crisis. It targets people at their most vulnerable—sick, scared, possibly dying—then adds financial catastrophe to their existing burdens. This is not healthcare; this is systematic cruelty dressed up in billing codes and collection calls.

The Pre-ACA vs. Post-ACA Reality

Before the Affordable Care Act was passed in 2010, health insurance functioned even worse than it does now. Insurance companies could deny coverage for pre-existing conditions, meaning a previous cancer diagnosis, or diabetes, or heart disease could make you permanently uninsurable. They could impose lifetime caps on coverage, cutting off benefits once you'd accumulated enough medical expenses—right when you needed insurance most. They could retroactively cancel your policy if you'd made any mistake on your application, and leave sick people suddenly uninsured and liable for bills they thought were covered.

The ACA eliminated these specific horrors. No more denials for pre-existing conditions. No more lifetime caps. No more rescission. Young adults could stay on their parents' insurance until age 26. Insurance plans had to cover preventive care without cost-sharing. These were real improvements that helped millions of people.

Yet medical bankruptcy rates haven't significantly decreased since the ACA's implementation.

This fact reveals something important about American healthcare's failures. The ACA fixed some problems while leaving the fundamental bankruptcy-generation mechanisms intact. High deductibles still transfer massive financial risk to patients. Coinsurance still requires people to pay 20% of hundred-thousand-dollar treatments. Narrow networks still leave patients vulnerable to surprise out-of-network bills. Insurance company denials still force patients to appeal or pay out of pocket. Meanwhile, the cost of care itself has continued rising faster than wages, making out-of-pocket burdens progressively less affordable even as coverage has expanded.

The ACA expanded coverage substantially. Millions gained insurance through Medicaid expansion in participating states and through subsidized marketplace plans. The uninsured rate dropped from about 16% to around 10% of non-elderly adults. By the conventional metric of "coverage percentage," the ACA succeeded, but coverage and protection are different things. The ACA increased the former without adequately ensuring the latter.

The marketplace plans illustrate this gap. Bronze plans—the cheapest option—have deductibles routinely exceeding $7,500 for individuals. Silver plans have deductibles of $4,000-$5,000. Even gold plans require $2,000-$3,000 in deductible spending. These deductibles would be bankrupting for any family earning median income or less, yet millions of Americans carry these plans because they're the most affordable options available or because their employers offer similar high-deductible plans.

The ACA included subsidies to make premiums affordable based on income, which helped many people purchase coverage they couldn't otherwise afford. The subsidies don't address deductibles and coinsurance, however. A family earning $60,000 might receive substantial premium subsidies but still face a $6,000 deductible and 20% coinsurance on everything after that. The subsidies help them buy inadequate insurance. They're still vulnerable to bankruptcy if they get seriously ill.

Employer-sponsored insurance—covering about 160 million Americans—has gotten worse since the ACA. Employers have responded to rising healthcare costs by shifting more expenses to employees through higher deductibles and larger coinsurance shares. The percentage of workers with deductibles of $1,000 or more has increased dramatically. Many now face deductibles of $3,000, $5,000, or even $8,000. These increases happened after the ACA passed, not before, as employers used healthcare reform as cover for reducing the value of coverage they provided.

The surprise billing crisis continued largely unabated until the No Surprises Act took effect in 2022—twelve years after the ACA passed. During that decade, millions of Americans with ACA-compliant insurance plans received surprise bills from out-of-network providers they never chose and couldn't avoid. The ACA did nothing to prevent this common path to medical debt and bankruptcy.

The No Surprises Act has helped reduce certain types of surprise billing, particularly for emergency services and ancillary providers such as anesthesiologists and radiologists. Still, significant gaps remain. Ground ambulances aren't covered by the law, leaving patients vulnerable to bills of $3,000 or more for ambulance transport they didn't choose and couldn't avoid. Some types of out-of-network care still generate surprise bills, and the law does nothing about the underlying problem: the massive cost-sharing that insurance plans require.

Even when surprise billing is eliminated and all providers are in network, patients with serious illnesses still face financial catastrophe. If your cancer treatment is billed at $300,000 and your insurance is ACA-compliant with a $6,000 deductible and 20% coinsurance, you still owe $66,000 out of pocket, depending on your insurer's out-of-pocket max. That's not a surprise bill. That's the system working exactly as designed, post-ACA. You're compliant with the individual mandate. Your insurance meets all ACA requirements. You followed all the rules. You're still bankrupt.

The ACA's consumer protections helped many people but didn't address the fundamental affordability crisis. Medical debt continued accumulating faster than people could pay. By 2020, 17.8% of Americans had medical debt in collections. One-fifth of insured adults aged 18-64 incurred unaffordable out-of-pocket costs in 2020, a decade after the ACA passed. Among Medicare beneficiaries—who have government insurance theoretically more comprehensive than private plans—average out-of-pocket costs were $5,460 in 2016, with half spending at least 12% of income on healthcare.

These numbers represent the post-ACA reality. Coverage expanded. Protections improved. Medical bankruptcy continued at catastrophic levels.

The gap between the ACA's promise and its delivery reveals the limitations of reform that preserves private insurance's fundamental structure. The ACA worked within the existing system—regulating insurance companies more strictly, subsidizing premiums for low-income people, expanding Medicaid. These were meaningful changes, but they didn't change the basic model where insurance companies profit by denying coverage, hospitals charge arbitrary prices, and patients bear catastrophic financial risk if they get seriously ill.

True protection from medical bankruptcy requires fundamentally restructuring how healthcare is financed—either through universal public insurance, heavily regulated private insurance with strict out-of-pocket caps (like Germany), or through some hybrid model. The ACA attempted to regulate private insurance into adequacy. It partially succeeded at expanding coverage. It failed to eliminate medical bankruptcy because it left the bankruptcy-generating mechanisms in place.

This isn't an argument that the ACA accomplished nothing. It helped millions of people. Children with pre-existing conditions can now get insurance. Young adults have more coverage options. Preventive care is more accessible. These matter. They just matter less than we'd hoped because the financial catastrophe of serious illness remains largely unchanged for people with insurance.

The ACA's failure to eliminate medical bankruptcy despite expanding coverage demonstrates that coverage alone isn't sufficient. You can mandate that everyone have insurance, subsidize premiums to make it affordable, require that insurance plans meet minimum standards, and still end up with a system that bankrupts hundreds of thousands of families annually. The problem isn't just lack of coverage. It's inadequate coverage, and that is profitable for insurance companies, which means the profit motive systematically undermines adequate protection.

Post-ACA medical bankruptcy looks remarkably similar to pre-ACA medical bankruptcy. The bills still arrive. The collections agencies still call. The lawsuits still happen. The wage garnishments continue. The credit scores tank. The families lose their homes. The only real difference is that now more of the people filing bankruptcy have insurance, because more people have insurance, period. The insurance they have isn't adequate to prevent bankruptcy, though, which means the ACA reformed American healthcare while leaving its most destructive feature fundamentally intact.

The System Working As Designed

There's a comforting story Americans tell themselves about medical bankruptcy: it's a tragic flaw in an otherwise well-intentioned system. An unfortunate side effect. A problem we're working on fixing. A bug, not a feature.

This story is false.

Medical bankruptcy isn't a system malfunction. It's a system output. American healthcare is specifically designed to extract maximum revenue from patients, insurance companies, and the government while distributing financial risk downward onto sick individuals and their families. Medical bankruptcy occurs when that risk distribution works exactly as intended.

Consider the flow of money: patients pay premiums to insurance companies. Insurance companies pay negotiated rates to hospitals and physicians. Hospitals pay staff and suppliers while maintaining profit margins or, for nonprofits, accumulating reserves. Everyone involved in providing or financing healthcare makes money—except the patient, who pays premiums while healthy and then pays again through deductibles and coinsurance when sick.

This model isn't designed to prevent medical bankruptcy. It's designed to profit from patients at every stage while using high cost-sharing to reduce insurance companies' payouts. The result is that patients bear catastrophic risk. When that risk materializes through serious illness, patients face catastrophic bills. When they can't pay those bills, they go bankrupt. This isn't a failure. It's the predictable outcome of a system that prioritizes profit over protection.

The insurance companies make money by collecting premiums and denying claims. Their profit margins improve when they pay out less in benefits, which creates a fundamental conflict of interest: they profit when you don't get the care you need. High deductibles serve this purpose beautifully. They mean the insurance company pays nothing until you've spent thousands out of pocket. For many patients, annual medical expenses never exceed the deductible, meaning the insurance company collected premiums and paid zero benefits. That's pure profit.

Even after you meet your deductible, coinsurance means you keep paying. Twenty percent of a $100,000 hospitalization is $20,000. The insurance company pays $80,000—a lot of money, but they've been collecting premiums from you for years. Over a lifetime, most people pay far more in premiums than they receive in benefits. The minority who get seriously ill and need expensive care face such high cost-sharing that they often can't afford treatment or go bankrupt trying. Either outcome is profitable for the insurance company: you either forgo expensive care, reducing their payouts, or you pay a huge chunk yourself, also reducing their payouts.

Hospitals make money through volume and price. More patients, higher prices, more profit. The "chargemaster" prices are deliberately inflated so that negotiated "discounts" still yield high margins. Hospitals have no incentive to reduce prices because doing so would reduce revenue. They have every incentive to maximize prices right up to the point where patients and insurance companies push back hard enough to threaten volume. That equilibrium point is well above what would be affordable for most patients, which is fine with hospitals because unpaid bills can be written off as charity care for tax purposes, sent to collections for partial recovery, or pursued through lawsuits and wage garnishment.

Pharmaceutical companies make money by charging whatever the market will bear, which in the U.S. means far more than they charge in other countries. A medication that costs $50 in Canada might cost $500 in the U.S. This isn't because American patients need higher-quality medications. It's because American drug pricing is largely unregulated, allowing pharmaceutical companies to charge based on desperation rather than cost. You can't negotiate when you need insulin to survive. You can't shop around when your oncologist prescribes a specific chemotherapy drug. You pay or you die. The pharmaceutical companies understand this. They price accordingly.

Every entity in the system profits from patient financial vulnerability. The sicker you are, the more money flows through the system—to hospitals, physicians, pharmaceutical companies, medical device manufacturers, and all the middlemen who've positioned themselves between patients and care. The only entity that loses money is you, the patient. When you can't lose any more money because you don't have any left, you file bankruptcy. The system has extracted everything it can extract. Now you're released, financially destroyed but no longer a source of revenue.

This explains why medical bankruptcy hasn't decreased despite reform efforts. The reforms don't change the fundamental profit extraction model. They just regulate it slightly, requiring certain consumer protections while preserving the underlying structure. As long as healthcare is organized around profit rather than around care, medical bankruptcy will continue because bankruptcy is what happens when profit extraction exceeds patient capacity to pay.

The moral obscenity of this system is profound. We're bankrupting people for the crime of getting sick. We're punishing cancer patients for having cancer. We're destroying families financially because someone needed medical care. We are doing this deliberately, and systemically, because it's profitable. Not profitable for patients, but profitable for the corporations that have captured American healthcare and turned it into a wealth extraction mechanism.

The 530,000 families filing medical bankruptcy annually aren't victims of a broken system. They're victims of a working system—a system designed to generate maximum profit by imposing maximum risk on patients. When you understand this, everything else makes sense: the arbitrary prices, the surprise bills, the insurance denials, the aggressive collections, the lawsuits against patients who qualify for charity care. It's all designed to extract money. When extraction reaches its limit—when patients literally cannot pay more—the system discards them through bankruptcy and moves on to the next cohort of patients with money or credit left to extract.

American healthcare isn't designed to prevent medical bankruptcy. It's designed to generate it as the inevitable endpoint when profit extraction exceeds financial capacity. The system works perfectly. It just doesn't work for patients. It works for everyone else—the insurance executives, the hospital administrators, the pharmaceutical companies, the investors, the shareholders. They all profit while patients go bankrupt.

That's not a bug. That's the feature.

> *"What if I just get filthy rich?" you say. Well, while our healthcare system fails to inoculate us against common disease, it also offers a robust defense against us chasing the American Dream.*

CHAPTER 7

The Entrepreneur's Trap

The Woman Who Couldn't Leave

The following scenario is a composite constructed from common patterns among would-be entrepreneurs trapped by employer-based insurance. The details are hypothetical, but the dynamics are widespread and documented.

Maria Sanchez was thirty-four years old when she realized she was going to spend the rest of her life working for someone else—not because she lacked talent or ambition, but because she had asthma.

She'd been managing a marketing department for a mid-sized company for six years. She was good at her job. Great at it, actually. Clients specifically requested to work with her. She'd built systems that doubled the department's efficiency. She'd trained three people who'd gone on to senior positions at other companies. Her boss knew she was underpaid and overworked. He also knew she wasn't going anywhere.

Because Maria had health insurance through her employer, and she needed health insurance reliably and continuously.

She'd had asthma since childhood—the kind that required daily controller medications, rescue inhalers for flare-ups, regular pulmonologist appointments, and quarterly breathing tests. Her asthma was generally well-controlled with medication, but she'd had three emergency room visits in the past five years when respiratory infections triggered severe attacks. Without her daily medications, her asthma would spiral out of control within days. Her controller inhaler alone cost $400 per month without insurance. With her employer's insurance, she paid $40. Add the rescue inhaler, pulmonologist visits, periodic chest X-rays, and allergy medications that helped prevent triggers, and her total monthly healthcare costs without insurance would exceed $800. With insurance, she paid around $150.

She'd been planning to start her own consulting business for three years. She had the expertise. She had the client relationships—former clients kept asking if she did freelance work. She had a business plan, startup capital saved, and a network ready to support her. She was ready to leave.

She just couldn't.

What prevented it was the fact that individual health insurance through the ACA marketplace would cost her $850 per month for a plan with a $7,000 deductible. That meant paying $10,200 in premiums annually plus another $7,000 in out-of-pocket costs before insurance covered anything beyond preventive care. Nearly $18,000 per year in healthcare costs—before making a single dollar of business profit.

Her employer-sponsored insurance cost her $200 per month in premiums with a $2,000 deductible. The employer subsidized the rest—about $600 per month that Maria never saw but absolutely depended on. Leaving her job meant losing that $600 monthly subsidy. It meant tripling her insurance costs at exactly the moment her income would become uncertain.

She ran the numbers repeatedly. To replace her current salary plus cover the increased insurance costs, her consulting business would need to generate $75,000 in its first year just to break even with her current situation. Possible, but risky. What if the business turned out to struggle in year one? If clients were slow to materialize? If income was inconsistent during the startup phase?

She couldn't risk a coverage gap. Her asthma required continuous medication—missing even a few days meant declining lung function and increased risk of severe attacks. She couldn't risk the marketplace plan's high deductible—what if she had a severe asthma attack requiring hospitalization during the year she was paying everything out-of-pocket? She couldn't risk the instability of marketplace coverage that might change networks annually, forcing her to find new pulmonologists and restart prior authorizations for her medications.

So she stayed. She stayed in a job that paid her $15,000 less than her market value. She stayed working for a boss who took credit for her ideas. She stayed watching less talented colleagues leave for better opportunities while she remained trapped. She stayed because American healthcare is designed to keep people like her employed by corporations rather than building their own businesses.

Her employer knew it. During her last salary negotiation, when she'd asked for a raise to match market rates, her boss had said, "You know the benefits here are really competitive. The healthcare alone is worth a lot." Translation: you can't leave because of your asthma, so why would I pay you more?

She was thirty-four years old with a chronic condition, exceptional skills, entrepreneurial ambition, and absolutely no path to self-employment that didn't involve risking her health and financial stability. She had golden handcuffs made of inhaler prescriptions and insurance networks. The American healthcare system had transformed her asthma into a mechanism of employment coercion.

This is what happens when healthcare is tied to employment. This is the trap. Maria wasn't alone—millions of Americans with chronic conditions, with families, with any healthcare needs that couldn't tolerate interruption, faced the same impossible choice: stay employed or risk losing access to care.

The entrepreneurial dreams, the business innovations, the economic dynamism—all sacrificed because American healthcare is designed to benefit employers who want captive workforces rather than workers who want the freedom to build something of their own.

How Healthcare Became Job Handcuffs

Healthcare wasn't always tied to employment in America. The connection emerged accidentally during World War II and became permanent because it served employer interests, not because it made sense as healthcare policy.

During the war, the federal government imposed wage controls to prevent inflation. Employers couldn't offer higher salaries to attract workers in a tight labor market. They needed another way to compete for talent. Someone realized that fringe benefits—including health insurance—weren't subject to wage controls. Employers could offer health insurance as a substitute for higher wages.

The IRS decided in 1943 that employer-paid health insurance wasn't taxable income to employees. This made employer-sponsored insurance tax-advantaged: employers could deduct the cost as a business expense, and employees didn't pay income tax on the value of the benefit. It was cheaper to compensate workers with health insurance than with equivalent salary.

This tax advantage was codified in 1954, making employer-sponsored insurance permanently advantaged over individual coverage. If your employer bought your insurance, it was tax-free. If you bought your own insurance, you paid with after-tax dollars. The tax code created a massive incentive for insurance to flow through employers rather than to individuals.

This wasn't healthcare policy. It was labor policy disguised as tax policy that gave employers enormous power over workers.

It worked because once healthcare was tied to employment, leaving your job meant losing your healthcare. This created dependency. Employees couldn't easily leave for better opportunities, couldn't negotiate from positions of strength, couldn't walk away from bad working conditions without risking their families' access to medical care.

Employers discovered that health insurance was an excellent retention tool. Offer decent health coverage and employees stay even when wages stagnate, working conditions deteriorate, or better opportunities exist elsewhere. The threat of losing healthcare keeps people in jobs they hate, tolerating treatment they shouldn't accept, forgoing opportunities they should pursue.

This effect is strongest for people who most need healthcare: people with chronic conditions, people with sick family members, older workers approaching Medicare age but not yet 65, and parents with children who need consistent pediatric care. These workers are trapped. They can't risk coverage gaps. They can't afford individual market premiums. They can't tolerate the instability of changing insurance networks. They stay employed regardless of whether the job serves their interests, because the alternative is losing access to healthcare.

As mentioned, this is called "job lock" in economic literature. It's well-documented. Studies show that employer-sponsored insurance significantly reduces labor mobility—people change jobs less frequently when losing health insurance is a consequence. They stay in jobs that don't match their skills. They don't relocate for better opportunities. They don't start businesses. They remain employed to maintain healthcare access, even when remaining employed means accepting lower wages, worse conditions, and limited career growth.

The system doesn't just fail to support entrepreneurship—it actively prevents it by design. Employer-based insurance was created to help employers retain workers during wartime labor shortages. It succeeded so well at creating employee dependency that it became permanent. Employers lobbied to preserve it. Unions negotiated for better employer-provided coverage rather than pushing for universal healthcare. The system entrenched itself.

Seventy years later, employer-based insurance covers about 150 million Americans—half the population. It's the dominant form of health coverage for working-age adults. It still functions exactly as originally designed: to give employers power over workers by controlling access to healthcare.

You can't leave your job without losing your healthcare. You can't negotiate aggressively for higher wages when your employer controls your access to medical care. You can't start a business when doing so means paying three to five times more for inferior individual coverage. You can't take career risks when healthcare access depends on maintaining continuous employment.

This isn't an unfortunate side effect of how we finance healthcare. It's the intended mechanism. Healthcare as employment coercion. Healthcare as golden handcuffs. Healthcare as a tool that benefits employers at the expense of workers' economic freedom and career mobility.

The trap isn't accidental. It's structural, deliberate, and designed to keep workers dependent on employers who control their access to care.

The Coverage Gap When You Leave Traditional Employment

Leaving a job that provides health insurance doesn't just mean finding new coverage—it means navigating a deliberately complex system designed to make continuous coverage difficult and expensive.

COBRA—the Consolidated Omnibus Budget Reconciliation Act—theoretically allows you to continue your employer-sponsored coverage for eighteen months after leaving a job. It sounds reasonable until you see the cost.

Under COBRA, you pay the full premium that your employer was paying plus a 2% administrative fee. That employer subsidy you never saw? It's gone. The $600 per month your employer was paying toward your insurance? Now you pay it.

For many people, this means COBRA premiums of $1,500 to $2,500 per month for family coverage. If you left your job to start a business, you're paying this while generating zero income during startup. If you were laid off, you're paying this while unemployed. If you quit because of hostile working conditions, you're paying this while job hunting. The people who most need affordable coverage during employment transitions are charged premiums they can't afford.

COBRA isn't really continuation coverage. It's a prohibitively expensive option that exists primarily so employers can claim they offered continuing coverage while knowing most people can't afford it. The continuation is theoretical. The coverage gap is real.

The alternative is the ACA marketplace. Individual coverage purchased through healthcare.gov or state exchanges, theoretically available to anyone, with income-based subsidies for people earning between 100% and 400% of the federal poverty level.

Theoretically.

In practice, marketplace coverage has significant problems for people leaving traditional employment.

First, the cost. Without the employer subsidy, you pay the full premium. For a forty-year-old individual, average marketplace premiums range from $450 to $600 per month depending on location and plan. For families, $1,200 to $1,800 per month is common. These are premiums alone—before deductibles, coinsurance, or out-of-pocket costs.

Second, the deductibles. Marketplace plans typically have high deductibles—$6,000 to $8,000 for individual coverage, $12,000 or more for family plans. You pay these amounts out-of-pocket before insurance covers anything beyond preventive care. For someone starting a business with uncertain income, a $7,000 deductible means the insurance you're paying $600 monthly for won't actually help until you've spent $7,000 on care.

Third, the instability. Marketplace plans change annually. Networks shift. Insurance carriers enter and exit markets. Premiums increase. Deductibles rise. You can't count on keeping the same plan or the same providers from year to year.

I know this personally. I purchase insurance through the ACA marketplace as a locums provider (in my case, as a nurse practitioner who works temporary, short-term assignments to fill staffing gaps in local clinics). The coverage has been okay, but I've had to change insurance carriers every couple of years—either because the premiums became unaffordable or because the carrier dropped coverage in my area entirely. Each time I switch carriers, I lose access to established providers, have to explain my medical history to new providers, and hope the new plan's network includes the doctors I need.

This instability is acceptable when you're healthy and rarely use healthcare. It's catastrophic when you have chronic conditions requiring continuity of care. Switching insurance annually means finding new specialists who accept the new plan, getting prior authorizations approved again, hoping your medications are covered by the new formulary, and rebuilding relationships with providers who don't know your history.

Fourth, the subsidy cliff. Income-based subsidies help some people afford marketplace coverage. But they're designed for stable, predictable income. If you're starting a business, your income fluctuates month to month. Earn too much one year and you lose subsidies retroactively, owing thousands in premium repayments at tax time. Earn too little and you might fall into the Medicaid coverage gap in states that haven't expanded.

Fifth, the coverage quality. Marketplace plans often have narrower networks than employer plans. Fewer doctors accept them. Fewer hospitals are in-network. You might find affordable premiums only to discover the plan doesn't include your current physicians or the specialists you need.

The result is that leaving employer coverage means either paying COBRA rates you can't afford or buying marketplace coverage that costs more, covers less, and provides less stability than the employer plan you're leaving. For someone starting a business, these costs come at exactly the wrong time—when income is uncertain and startup costs are high.

Real math: to replace a typical employer health insurance subsidy, a new business needs to generate an additional $7,000 to $10,000 annually just to break even on healthcare costs. That's revenue that doesn't go to business growth, equipment, hiring, or the entrepreneur's salary. That's revenue that exists solely to make up for the employer subsidy you lost by leaving traditional employment.

This isn't a minor inconvenience. It's a significant economic barrier to entrepreneurship, career changes, and labor mobility. It keeps people employed when they'd be better off starting businesses. It keeps talented people in jobs that don't use their skills because leaving means unaffordable healthcare costs.

The coverage gap when you leave traditional employment isn't accidental. It's designed into a system that ties healthcare to jobs, subsidizes employer coverage through tax policy, and makes individual coverage substantially more expensive. The gap serves employer interests by keeping workers employed. It harms workers by limiting their economic freedom and career options.

The Medicaid Coverage Gap

In states that refused to expand Medicaid under the ACA, there's a literal coverage gap where people earn too much for Medicaid but too little for marketplace subsidies. These people have no coverage option at all.

Pre-ACA, Medicaid covered low-income children, pregnant women, elderly people, and people with disabilities. Most states didn't cover non-disabled, non-pregnant adults regardless of how poor they were. A single adult earning poverty wages working at Walmart had no Medicaid eligibility and couldn't afford individual insurance. They remained uninsured.

The ACA was designed to fix this by expanding Medicaid to cover all adults with incomes up to 138% of the federal poverty level—about $20,000 for an individual, $41,000 for a family of four. The federal government would pay 90% of the cost. States would expand coverage to millions of previously uninsured low-income adults.

Then the Supreme Court made expansion optional. Ten states refused to expand. These states—concentrated in the South, with large Black populations—chose to leave their poorest residents uninsured rather than accept federal funding that would primarily help people of color.

This created the coverage gap. In non-expansion states, Medicaid still covers only the pre-ACA populations: children, pregnant women, elderly, disabled. A single adult earning $15,000 per year doesn't qualify for Medicaid (too healthy, wrong demographics) and doesn't qualify for marketplace subsidies (which start at 100% of federal poverty level, approximately $15,650). They fall into the gap: too poor for subsidized marketplace coverage, ineligible for Medicaid.

This affects exactly the people trying to start small businesses. Self-employed income is variable and often low in the early years. A freelancer earning $12,000 one year might earn $18,000 the next. In non-expansion states, they cycle between having no coverage option when income is low and barely qualifying for subsidized marketplace plans when income rises slightly.

The administrative nightmare of this instability is crushing. Medicaid eligibility requires monthly income verification. If you earn more than expected one month, you lose Medicaid mid-year. If you earn less than expected, you might retroactively qualify but have to reapply and document income changes. Switching between Medicaid and marketplace coverage means changing provider networks, reauthorizing prescriptions, and hoping your doctors accept whichever insurance you happen to qualify for that month.

For entrepreneurs with variable income, this makes planning impossible. You don't know which insurance you'll have or whether you'll have any insurance at all. You can't maintain continuity with providers. You can't budget healthcare costs because they fluctuate wildly based on which coverage category you fall into month to month.

The coverage gap disproportionately affects Black and Brown entrepreneurs in Southern non-expansion states. These are states that refused Medicaid expansion specifically because expansion would primarily help Black residents. The coverage gap is racist policy by design—deliberately leaving poor Black and Brown people uninsured while claiming fiscal responsibility.

The people in the coverage gap are working. They're just earning poverty wages at jobs that don't provide insurance or they're self-employed in the early stages of building businesses. They need healthcare. They have no way to get it. They remain uninsured not because they're lazy or gaming the system but because their states deliberately chose to exclude them from both Medicaid and marketplace subsidies.

This is particularly cruel for entrepreneurs. Starting a business often means low or variable income in the first years. In expansion states, Medicaid covers you during the startup phase when income is low. In non-expansion states, you have no coverage. You're forced to choose between seeking healthcare you need and paying out-of-pocket costs you can't afford, or avoiding care and hoping you stay healthy until your business generates enough income to afford marketplace premiums.

The coverage gap kills entrepreneurship among exactly the populations who most need economic opportunities. Poor people trying to build businesses in states that refuse Medicaid expansion face an impossible situation: no coverage when income is low, unaffordable coverage when income rises slightly, and no stability anywhere in between.

This serves no policy purpose except cruelty and control. It doesn't save money—uninsured people still get sick, still need care, still end up in emergency rooms generating uncompensated costs that get passed to everyone else. It exists purely to punish poor people and prevent them from accessing the healthcare coverage that would help them build economic stability.

How This Stifles Innovation and Business Creation

The connection between healthcare and entrepreneurship isn't speculative—it's documented, quantified, and economically significant. Tying healthcare to employment reduces business formation, stifles innovation, and costs the economy billions in unrealized economic activity.

Entrepreneurship requires risk-taking. You leave stable employment with predictable income for uncertain prospects of building something new. You invest time and capital before seeing returns. You accept the possibility of failure in exchange for the possibility of success. This is healthy economic risk-taking that drives innovation, creates jobs, and generates economic growth.

The consequence is that you can't take these risks when losing healthcare. Healthcare needs don't pause while you build a business. Chronic conditions require continuous management. Children need pediatric care. Families can't tolerate gaps in coverage. The risk of entrepreneurship becomes unacceptable when it includes the risk of losing access to medical care.

How many businesses were never started because healthcare was tied to employment? We can't know exactly, but research provides estimates. Studies show that employer-sponsored insurance reduces entrepreneurship by 25-50% among people with chronic health conditions or family members with high healthcare needs. That's not a small effect—that's half of potential businesses never getting started because health insurance was employer-provided rather than universally available.

The economic cost compounds. Each business not started is jobs not created, innovations not developed, economic activity not generated. Multiply this across millions of would-be entrepreneurs over decades and the economic loss is staggering. How many breakthrough innovations died because the person who conceived them couldn't risk leaving employer coverage? How many small businesses that would have employed dozens or hundreds of people never existed because the founder had diabetes or a child with asthma?

The innovation loss is particularly severe in specific populations:

People with chronic conditions are effectively locked out of entrepreneurship. Diabetes, multiple sclerosis, rheumatoid arthritis, Crohn's disease, lupus—any condition requiring ongoing specialist care and expensive medications makes leaving employer coverage prohibitively risky. These people might have brilliant business ideas, exceptional skills, and strong entrepreneurial drive. They can't pursue it because their health conditions make individual insurance either unavailable (pre-ACA) or unaffordable (post-ACA).

Parents face the same trap. Children need consistent pediatric care, vaccinations, emergency coverage for injuries and illnesses. Leaving employer coverage means finding marketplace plans that include your children's current pediatricians, cover their prescriptions, and won't change networks mid-year forcing you to find new doctors. The instability is manageable when you're healthy and single. It's unacceptable when you're responsible for children's healthcare.

Older workers in their 50s and early 60s face the pre-Medicare gap. Medicare doesn't start until 65. Leaving employer coverage at 55 or 60 means a decade of buying individual coverage during the years when health typically declines and insurance costs rise. Marketplace premiums for people in their 60s can exceed $2,000 monthly. This makes entrepreneurship financially impossible for experienced workers in their peak earning years who should be starting businesses based on decades of industry expertise.

Anyone who's ever been seriously ill fears coverage denial or unaffordable premiums in the individual market. Even with ACA protections against pre-existing condition exclusions, people who've had cancer, heart attacks, strokes, or other serious illnesses know their healthcare costs will be high. They can't risk losing employer coverage that shields them from the full cost of ongoing monitoring, follow-up care, and treatment of complications.

Each of these populations includes people who could and would start businesses if healthcare weren't tied to employment. The skills, ambition, and business opportunities exist. What's missing is the ability to take entrepreneurial risk without simultaneously risking healthcare access.

The economic literature calls this "entrepreneurship lock"—the reduction in business formation caused by employer-based health insurance. It's particularly strong in the United States compared to countries with universal healthcare. Canada, the UK, France, Germany, and other countries with universal systems show higher rates of entrepreneurship in many sectors specifically because healthcare isn't tied to employment.

When a Canadian considers starting a business, healthcare doesn't factor into the decision. They keep their healthcare coverage whether employed or self-employed. When an American considers the same decision, healthcare is often the determining factor. Can I afford marketplace premiums? What if I have a health emergency during the first year? What happens to my children's coverage? The healthcare questions often kill the business idea before it starts.

This is a massive drag on American economic dynamism. The United States supposedly values entrepreneurship, innovation, and economic freedom. The healthcare system actively suppresses all three by making entrepreneurship contingent on either being wealthy enough to self-fund insurance or healthy enough to risk coverage gaps.

Large corporations benefit enormously from this arrangement. They face less competition from startups because potential founders can't afford to leave corporate employment. They retain talented employees who would otherwise start competing businesses. They can offer lower wages because healthcare coverage is valuable and alternatives are expensive. They can maintain market dominance because the barrier to entry isn't just building a better product—it's also affording health insurance during the startup phase.

The system is working exactly as designed. Not to promote innovation and entrepreneurship—to suppress it. Not to enable economic freedom—to limit it. Not to serve workers—to benefit the large employers who want to keep workers dependent and competition minimal.

The Gig Economy Trap

The rise of the gig economy over the past fifteen years demonstrates exactly how employer-based insurance gets exploited to avoid providing healthcare to workers.

Uber, Lyft, DoorDash, Instacart, TaskRabbit, and dozens of other platforms classify workers as independent contractors rather than employees. This classification is deliberate, legally contested, and enormously profitable for the platforms.

If gig workers were employees, platforms would have to provide health insurance (for workers exceeding 30 hours weekly under the ACA), pay employer-side payroll taxes, cover workers' compensation insurance, and comply with minimum wage and overtime laws. Classifying workers as independent contractors eliminates all these obligations. The platforms avoid costs. Workers bear all the risks.

The result: millions of gig workers earning poverty wages with no employer-provided healthcare. They're expected to buy individual coverage on marketplace exchanges with income insufficient to afford it.

Let's do the math for a full-time Uber driver. After vehicle expenses (gas, maintenance, insurance, depreciation), many drivers net $12-18 per hour. Working 40 hours weekly, that's roughly $25,000-37,000 annually. Marketplace insurance premiums for a single adult might be $400-600 monthly ($4,800-7,200 annually), with a deductible of $6,000-7,000. Total healthcare costs could reach $11,000-14,000 before insurance pays for anything beyond preventive care.

A gig worker earning $30,000 annually would pay over one-third of their income for health insurance that doesn't cover anything until they've spent another $6,000 out-of-pocket. This is financially impossible. So gig workers remain uninsured or underinsured, avoiding care, delaying treatment, and hoping they don't get seriously ill.

The platforms profit from this arrangement. By misclassifying employees as contractors, they avoid providing health insurance that would cost them thousands per worker annually. They can pay lower effective wages because they're not covering benefits. They shift all healthcare risk to workers who can least afford it.

This is deliberately designed exploitation. The platforms didn't accidentally classify workers wrong—they built their entire business model on avoiding the costs and obligations of being employers. The worker flexibility that platforms tout as an advantage is actually economic insecurity with no safety net. The freedom to set your own hours is the freedom to work as many hours as necessary to afford basic necessities while still not being able to afford healthcare.

If gig workers were classified as employees, which many should be based on the level of control platforms exercise over their work, the platforms would have to provide health insurance. Workers would have employer-subsidized coverage. The current system where gig workers buy individual coverage at full cost while earning poverty wages would end.

Platforms therefore lobby aggressively against employee classification. They spend millions on ballot initiatives and legislation to preserve their right to classify workers as contractors. They know that reclassifying workers as employees would fundamentally change their economics. They'd have to provide healthcare. They'd have to pay more. Their business models depend on exploiting workers by avoiding employment obligations.

California's Proposition 22 in 2020 exemplifies this. Uber, Lyft, and DoorDash spent $200 million—the most expensive ballot initiative in state history—to exempt themselves from a law that would have classified their workers as employees. They won. California gig workers remain independent contractors with no employer healthcare obligation.

The $200 million the platforms spent to avoid classifying workers as employees tells you exactly how valuable the misclassification is. That's how much it's worth to them to avoid providing health insurance and other benefits. They'd rather spend $200 million on one election than provide healthcare to their workers.

The gig economy trap is employer-based insurance weaponized. The platforms benefit from a system where health insurance flows through employers—by ensuring they're not legally employers, they avoid providing it. Workers are left buying individual coverage at full cost on income insufficient to afford it. The platforms extract value from workers' labor while shirking the healthcare costs that traditional employers bear.

This is only possible because healthcare is tied to employment in the first place. If the United States had universal healthcare, gig worker classification wouldn't determine healthcare access. Workers would have coverage whether employed, self-employed, or working for platforms that misclassify them as contractors. The platforms would lose their biggest cost advantage from misclassification. Workers would have healthcare security regardless of how their work was classified.

Instead, we have millions of gig workers in the coverage gap—earning too much for Medicaid in most states, earning too little to afford marketplace coverage, and working for platforms that deliberately avoid classifying them as employees to escape healthcare obligations. The gig economy didn't create this problem. It exploited a vulnerability created by tying healthcare to employment and then refusing to classify workers as employees.

The Pre-ACA Nightmare

Before the Affordable Care Act took effect in 2014, leaving employer coverage meant facing an individual insurance market that could deny coverage for any health history more serious than a common cold.

Had diabetes? Denied.

Had cancer, even years in remission? Denied.

Had depression or anxiety? Denied.

Had ever been pregnant? Denied as a pre-existing condition.

Had high blood pressure? Denied or charged premiums double the standard rate.

Had asthma? Denied or excluded from coverage for anything respiratory.

The individual insurance market pre-ACA operated on medical underwriting—insurers evaluated each applicant's health history and either denied coverage, charged higher premiums, excluded coverage for specific conditions, or imposed waiting periods before covering pre-existing conditions. This meant that anyone with significant health history was effectively locked out of individual coverage.

For people with chronic conditions, this made entrepreneurship impossible. If you had Type 1 diabetes, you couldn't leave employer coverage and start a business. There was no individual insurance available. You either stayed employed to maintain coverage or you went uninsured. Those were the only options.

The trap was complete and permanent. Once you had a serious health condition, you were locked into employer coverage for life. Leave your job and you'd never get individual insurance. This wasn't theoretical—this was documented, widespread practice by every major insurance carrier.

Rescission was even more insidious. You'd buy individual insurance, pay premiums for years, then get sick with something expensive like cancer. The insurance company would review your original application looking for any error or omission—did you forget to mention you'd taken antibiotics for a sinus infection five years ago? Did you fail to disclose that your doctor once suggested you might have high cholesterol? The insurer would use any discrepancy, no matter how minor, to retroactively cancel your coverage for "material misrepresentation." You'd be stuck with hundreds of thousands in medical bills for care you thought was insured.

This happened routinely. Congressional investigations found that insurers had entire departments dedicated to finding reasons to rescind coverage of expensive patients. They profited by collecting premiums from healthy people and canceling coverage when people got sick.

High-risk pools theoretically existed for people who couldn't get individual coverage, but only sixteen states had them pre-ACA, coverage was severely limited, premiums were astronomical, and waiting lists were common. They weren't real solutions—they were fig leaves allowing states to claim they addressed the uninsurable while actually leaving most people without options.

I have pre-existing conditions that would have excluded me from individual insurance coverage before the ACA—or at minimum, would have raised my premiums significantly enough to make coverage unaffordable. This isn't unusual. Most everyone has something that required follow-up at one point in time. The individual insurance market treated all of these as grounds for denial or premium increases.

The pre-ACA system created absolute job lock for anyone with health history. You couldn't start a business. You couldn't become self-employed. You couldn't leave corporate employment even if you were miserable, underpaid, or had a brilliant business idea. Your health history made you permanently dependent on employer coverage.

The ACA eliminated pre-existing condition exclusions in 2014. Insurers can no longer deny coverage, charge higher premiums, or exclude conditions from coverage based on health history. This was transformative. People with diabetes, cancer histories, depression, and every other previously excluded condition could finally buy individual insurance.

But—and this is critical—the ACA only solved the denial problem. It didn't solve the cost problem.

Individual insurance is still far more expensive than employer coverage because you pay the full premium instead of the employer-subsidized portion. The ACA made coverage available but not necessarily affordable. You can't be denied anymore, but you might not be able to afford the $800 monthly premium even though you're legally entitled to buy it.

So the trap loosened but didn't disappear. Pre-ACA, people with health conditions couldn't get individual coverage at any price. Post-ACA, they can get coverage but often can't afford it. This is progress—significant progress. It's also still inadequate. The door isn't locked anymore, but it's expensive to walk through, and what's on the other side is coverage with high deductibles, narrow networks, and annual instability.

For would-be entrepreneurs with health conditions, the ACA expanded what was possible. You can start a business now without being completely locked out of coverage. You're still paying dramatically more than you were under employer insurance, though, often for coverage that's worse. The entrepreneurship tax for having health conditions decreased but didn't disappear.

The Financial Reality of Individual Coverage

Even with ACA protections eliminating pre-existing condition denials, the financial reality of individual coverage makes entrepreneurship difficult and often prohibitively expensive.

Average marketplace premiums for a forty-year-old individual range from $450 to $600 per month depending on location and plan tier. That's $5,400 to $7,200 annually in premiums. This is before the deductible—the amount you pay out-of-pocket before insurance covers anything.

Typical marketplace plan deductibles run $6,000 to $8,000 for individual coverage. Bronze plans have lower premiums but deductibles often exceed $8,000. Silver plans have moderate premiums and deductibles around $6,000-7,000. Gold plans have higher premiums but lower deductibles around $3,000-4,000. The fundamental trade-off remains: pay more monthly or pay more when you actually use care.

For family coverage, the numbers multiply. Average marketplace premiums for family plans run $1,200 to $1,800 monthly—$14,400 to $21,600 annually. Family deductibles typically range from $12,000 to $14,000. Out-of-pocket maximums reach $18,000+.

Let's make this concrete with an example. A thirty-eight-year-old woman starting a consulting business needs to buy individual coverage. She chooses a Silver plan at $550 per month with a $7,000 deductible. Her annual costs:

- Premiums: $6,600
- Deductible (assuming she uses any significant care): $7,000
- Total: $13,600 before insurance pays for anything beyond preventive care

If she has a health emergency—appendicitis, broken bone, pneumonia requiring hospitalization—she'll hit her deductible and potentially her out-of-pocket maximum (typically $9,000-9,500 for individual coverage). Her total annual costs could reach $15,000-16,000.

Compare this to employer coverage. When she was employed, she paid perhaps $200 per month in premiums ($2,400 annually) with a $2,000 deductible. Her maximum annual costs were around $4,400. Her employer was subsidizing roughly $600 per month ($7,200 annually) in additional premium costs she never saw.

Leaving employment to start her business means her healthcare costs increase from $4,400 annually to potentially $15,000+. That's an additional $10,000-11,000 in annual costs her business must generate just to maintain the same coverage she had as an employee.

This is the entrepreneurship tax. The additional cost of healthcare when you leave employer coverage and buy individual insurance. For healthy young people, it might be $3,000-4,000 annually. For older workers, people with chronic conditions, or families with children, it can reach $15,000-25,000 annually.

Starting a business requires capital. You need money for equipment, inventory, marketing, legal fees, accounting, website development, and dozens of other startup costs. Adding $10,000-20,000 in additional annual healthcare costs on top of these business expenses makes entrepreneurship accessible only to people with substantial savings or access to capital.

Real example: a mid-career professional in her forties wants to leave corporate employment and start a consulting practice. She's excellent at what she does, has client relationships ready to transfer, and has saved $30,000 for startup costs and living expenses during the first year.

Her employer currently subsidizes about $8,000 annually in health insurance costs. Leaving means she pays that $8,000 herself. Her $30,000 in savings now needs to cover:

- Living expenses: $15,000 (six months at reduced spending)
- Business startup costs: $8,000 (website, legal, marketing, equipment)
- Healthcare: $8,000 (individual marketplace coverage)
- Buffer: $-1,000 (she's already over budget)

She doesn't have enough saved. She needs another $5,000-10,000 just to cover the healthcare cost increase from leaving employer coverage. Unless she can generate revenue immediately, she can't afford to start her business.

This scenario repeats millions of times. Talented people with solid business ideas who can't afford to leave employer coverage because individual insurance costs consume the capital they need for business startup.

The income-based subsidies theoretically help some people. If you earn between 100% and 400% of the federal poverty level (roughly $15,000-$60,000 for an individual), you qualify for premium tax credits that reduce monthly costs. The catch is that these subsidies disappear at higher incomes, creating cliff effects where earning slightly more means losing thousands in subsidies.

For entrepreneurs with variable income, subsidy cliffs create nightmare scenarios. Earn more than expected during your first business year and you'll owe subsidy repayments at tax time—potentially thousands of dollars you weren't expecting. Underestimate your income and you miss out on subsidies you qualified for. The complexity makes planning impossible.

Furthermore, the coverage you're buying with these expensive premiums is often inferior to employer coverage. Marketplace plans typically have narrower networks—fewer doctors, fewer hospitals, more restrictions. Your current specialists might not accept marketplace plans. The hospital where you've been treated might be out-of-network. You might have to find entirely new providers just because you left employer coverage.

This is the financial reality: individual coverage costs 3-5 times more than the subsidized portion of employer coverage, covers less, offers less stability, and creates planning nightmares for anyone with variable income. These aren't minor inconveniences. They're massive economic barriers that prevent entrepreneurship, reduce labor mobility, and keep talented people employed in jobs that don't use their skills simply because affording healthcare any other way is impossible.

How Other Countries Enable Entrepreneurship

The connection between universal healthcare and entrepreneurship isn't theoretical—it's demonstrated in every developed country that's implemented universal coverage.

In Canada, starting a business doesn't mean losing healthcare. Every Canadian has provincial health insurance regardless of employment status. Entrepreneurs keep their coverage whether self-employed, employed, or unemployed. Healthcare access doesn't factor into the decision to start a business because it doesn't change based on employment.

This matters economically. Canada shows higher rates of self-employment than the United States in several sectors. While multiple factors influence entrepreneurship rates, healthcare is consistently cited as an advantage for Canadian entrepreneurs. They can take business risks without simultaneously risking healthcare access.

The United Kingdom's National Health Service provides coverage to every resident regardless of employment status. You don't lose NHS coverage when you leave a job. You don't pay more for coverage when self-employed. Starting a business means zero change in healthcare access. This removes a major barrier to entrepreneurship that American workers face.

France's healthcare system covers all residents with minimal out-of-pocket costs. Self-employed workers have the same coverage as employees. Healthcare financing is separate from employment status. French entrepreneurs don't calculate healthcare costs when deciding whether to start businesses—coverage is guaranteed regardless.

Germany, Japan, Australia, New Zealand, and virtually every developed country besides the United States has separated healthcare from employment. The specific mechanisms vary—some are single-payer systems, others are multi-payer with strong regulation—but they share a common feature: you don't lose healthcare coverage by leaving traditional employment.

The result is that entrepreneurship is less risky in countries with universal healthcare. You can start a business knowing you'll maintain healthcare access. You can take calculated business risks without simultaneously gambling with your health coverage. You can leave employment that doesn't serve your interests without abandoning access to medical care.

Research comparing entrepreneurship across countries consistently finds that universal healthcare facilitates business creation. Countries with national health systems show higher rates of entrepreneurship among populations with chronic health conditions, among older workers, and among parents with children—exactly the populations most locked into employer coverage in the United States.

The United States has lower self-employment rates than many peer countries despite supposedly valuing entrepreneurship and innovation. Americans talk about entrepreneurship more than we enable it. We celebrate startup culture while maintaining a healthcare system that makes starting businesses prohibitively risky for anyone with healthcare needs.

Countries with universal healthcare enable entrepreneurship by removing the healthcare penalty for leaving employment. Innovation happens when people can take risks. Universal healthcare makes risk-taking possible by ensuring that healthcare access doesn't depend on maintaining traditional employment.

The economic benefits compound. More entrepreneurship means more business formation, more job creation, more innovation, more economic dynamism. Some of these businesses fail—entrepreneurship always involves failure—but some succeed, and go on to create jobs, develop innovations, and drive economic growth. Countries with universal healthcare capture these benefits by making entrepreneurship accessible to anyone with good business ideas, not just people wealthy enough or healthy enough to afford healthcare independently.

The United States leaves this economic potential unrealized. We trap talented people in jobs they should leave, preventing business formation that would create jobs and drive innovation. We sacrifice economic dynamism to preserve a system that benefits large employers who want captive workforces.

This is a policy choice, not an inevitability. We could separate healthcare from employment as every other developed country has done. We could make entrepreneurship accessible to people with chronic conditions, parents with children, and older workers with decades of expertise. We could enable the innovation and business creation we claim to value.

Instead, we maintain employer-based insurance that functions as employment coercion, prevents entrepreneurship, and stifles the economic freedom and dynamism the system supposedly promotes.

The Employer Perspective: Why They Like This System

Employers didn't create the employer-based insurance system, but once it emerged they recognized its value and fought to preserve it. Because tying healthcare to employment gives employers enormous power over workers.

Employee retention improves dramatically when losing your job means losing healthcare. Workers stay longer at jobs they dislike. They tolerate worse working conditions. They accept lower wages. They remain employed even when better opportunities exist elsewhere because leaving means risking healthcare access for themselves and their families.

This is valuable to employers. High turnover costs money—recruiting, training, lost productivity while new employees get up to speed. Healthcare-dependent employees reduce turnover without employers having to improve wages, working conditions, or management quality. The threat of losing healthcare keeps employees in place.

The retention effect is particularly strong for employees with healthcare needs. Workers with chronic conditions can't risk coverage gaps. Parents can't risk their children losing pediatric care. Older workers can't risk the pre-Medicare gap. These employees become locked to their employers not by loyalty or satisfaction but by healthcare dependency.

Employers can leverage this. Wage negotiations go differently when employers control healthcare access. An employee asking for a raise can be reminded that the benefits package, particularly health insurance, is valuable. The implicit message: you can't get this anywhere else, so be grateful for what you have and stop asking for more.

The power dynamic is explicit for employees with chronic conditions or family members with high healthcare needs. Employers know these workers can't easily leave. They can offer lower wages, demand more hours, impose worse conditions, while knowing the employee is trapped. Threaten their job and you threaten their healthcare. That's leverage.

Employers also benefit from healthcare costs being largely invisible to employees. When employers pay $600 monthly toward an employee's insurance premium, the employee sees only the $200 they contribute from their paycheck. The other $600 disappears into "benefits." Employees don't see the full cost, so they undervalue it in compensation negotiations. Employers can offer lower wages by pointing to benefits employees don't fully appreciate.

The tax advantages amplify these benefits. Employer-paid health insurance is tax-deductible as a business expense and tax-free to employees. This makes health insurance a more tax-efficient form of compensation than salary. Employers save on payroll taxes. Employees avoid income tax on the value of coverage. The tax code subsidizes employer-based insurance, making it cheaper for employers to provide than equivalent salary increases.

Corporate lobbying to preserve employer-based insurance is substantial and consistent. The U.S. Chamber of Commerce, Business Roundtable, and major industry associations oppose universal healthcare proposals that would eliminate employer-based coverage. They frame this opposition as protecting quality and choice, but the underlying motivation is preserving employer power over workers.

Why would employers support universal healthcare? It would eliminate a major retention tool. Workers could leave without losing healthcare. Wage negotiations would change when employers couldn't point to health benefits as justification for lower salaries. The leverage employers currently have over healthcare-dependent workers would disappear.

Some employers—particularly small businesses that struggle to afford group coverage—would benefit from universal healthcare by no longer having to provide insurance. On the other hand, large corporations with comprehensive benefits packages would lose the competitive advantage those benefits provide in recruiting and retaining workers.

The system works for employers exactly as designed. It wasn't created for their benefit, but it benefits them enormously. They gain employee retention, wage leverage, reduced turnover, and power over workers who can't leave without losing healthcare. They gain all this while having healthcare costs partially subsidized through tax advantages.

Employees pay for this in reduced wages (because compensation goes to benefits rather than salary), reduced mobility (can't leave for better opportunities), reduced negotiating power (can't credibly threaten to leave), and reduced entrepreneurship (can't start businesses without losing coverage).

The employer-based system is working perfectly—for employers. It keeps workers dependent, reduces labor mobility, suppresses wages, prevents entrepreneurship that would compete with established corporations, and maintains power dynamics favorable to employers at workers' expense.

This is why employers fight to preserve it. Not because it's the best healthcare system—it demonstrably isn't. But because it's the best system for maintaining employer power over workers. That power is valuable enough to justify lobbying millions annually to prevent the universal healthcare that would eliminate it.

The Psychological Toll

The financial barriers to entrepreneurship created by employer-based insurance are quantifiable. The psychological toll is harder to measure, but equally real.

Fear of leaving employment permeates career decisions for anyone with healthcare needs. You see opportunities you can't pursue. You have business ideas you can't execute. You watch younger, healthier people take risks you'd take in a heartbeat if healthcare weren't tied to your job. The fear isn't irrational—losing healthcare access is genuinely dangerous. But watching your potential go unrealized because of a healthcare system design is limiting, constraining, and soul-crushing.

Dreams get deferred indefinitely. "Maybe when the kids are grown." "Maybe when I qualify for Medicare." "Maybe when I've saved more." It's just that the savings threshold keeps moving because healthcare costs keep rising. The timeline stretches. "Someday" becomes never. The business you wanted to start, the career change you wanted to make, the self-employment you craved—all abandoned not because you lacked ability but because you couldn't risk losing healthcare.

Resentment builds. You watch people without health conditions leave jobs and start businesses. You read success stories about entrepreneurs who took the leap. You know you could do it too. You're trapped anyway. The resentment isn't directed at the successful entrepreneurs—it's directed at a system that makes success contingent on being healthy enough to risk coverage gaps.

The "what ifs" multiply. What if you'd started that business ten years ago? What if you'd pursued that idea when you first had it? What if you weren't locked into employment by health insurance? You can't know what would have happened, but you know what didn't happen because healthcare was tied to your job. The unrealized potential haunts you.

Chronic stress from healthcare insecurity affects mental health even for people who remain employed. You worry about losing your job—not just for the income loss but for the healthcare loss. You tolerate bad management because leaving means unaffordable insurance. You stay in toxic work environments because healthcare for your child with asthma depends on maintaining employment. The constant low-level stress of healthcare dependency takes a toll.

The trapped feeling erodes autonomy and dignity. You're not choosing to stay at your job because you love it or because it's the best use of your skills. You're staying because leaving means losing healthcare. This isn't voluntary employment—it's coerced employment with healthcare access as the coercion mechanism. You know you're trapped. Your employer knows you're trapped. The system is designed to trap you. That knowledge is psychologically corrosive.

For people who do leave employment to start businesses despite the healthcare barriers, the stress of insurance instability continues. You're paying dramatically more for worse coverage. You're changing plans annually because carriers exit markets or premiums spike. You're hoping nothing serious happens because your deductible is $8,000. You're constantly calculating whether you can afford to see doctors or whether you should wait and hope problems resolve on their own.

The psychological burden isn't evenly distributed. Healthy young people experience less stress because they use less healthcare and have more coverage options. People with chronic conditions, parents with children, older workers, and anyone with significant health history bear the full psychological weight of navigating a system designed to make their healthcare access contingent on employment status.

The impact extends to families. Parents make career decisions based on which parent's employer provides better health insurance, not which career better utilizes their skills or provides better income. Families plan around insurance coverage—you can't change jobs during pregnancy, can't leave employment when children have ongoing specialist care, can't risk coverage gaps when family members have chronic conditions.

The mental health cost is substantial and unacknowledged. How many people are depressed, anxious, or burned out specifically because healthcare dependency traps them in jobs that don't serve them? How many people suffer chronic stress from healthcare insecurity despite being employed? How many people experience the psychological damage of knowing their potential will go unrealized because they can't risk losing healthcare?

These costs don't appear in economic analyses of employer-based insurance. They're not quantified in studies comparing healthcare systems. But they're real, widespread, and directly caused by tying healthcare to employment. The psychological toll of healthcare dependency is a tax Americans pay for a system designed to benefit employers at workers' expense.

The System Working As Designed

Employer-based health insurance appears to be an accident of history—something that emerged during World War II wage controls and persisted through inertia and tax policy, but its persistence isn't accidental. It continues because it serves powerful interests despite harming workers, entrepreneurs, and economic dynamism.

As mentioned, the system wasn't designed for employee benefit. It emerged as an employer recruitment tool during wartime labor shortages, was made permanent through tax advantages that benefited both employers and insurers, and evolved into a mechanism of employment coercion that gives employers power over workers by controlling access to healthcare.

This serves corporate interests perfectly. Large employers get employee retention without improving wages or working conditions.

- They get leverage in negotiations by controlling healthcare access.
- They get reduced competition from startups because potential founders can't afford to leave employment.
- They get a captive workforce dependent on maintaining jobs to maintain healthcare.

Insurance companies benefit by having employers as large, stable customers instead of dealing with millions of individual purchasers. Administrative costs are lower when selling to large employer groups. Risk pools are better when enrollment is mandatory through employment rather than voluntary in individual markets. The employer-based system provides insurance companies with guaranteed, stable business.

The system harms workers by limiting labor mobility, reducing wages (because compensation goes to benefits rather than salary), preventing entrepreneurship, and creating healthcare dependency that employers leverage for retention and control. It harms the economy by stifling business formation, reducing labor market efficiency, and preventing innovation that would occur if talented people could start businesses without risking healthcare access.

It's just that the harms to workers and the economy are diffuse and hard to quantify precisely. The benefits to employers and insurers are concentrated and clear. So the system persists despite being economically inefficient and morally indefensible, because the entities with power to change it benefit from maintaining it.

Tying healthcare to employment serves no healthcare purpose. It doesn't improve health outcomes. It doesn't reduce costs. It doesn't increase access to care. It exists purely to benefit employers who want dependent workers and insurers who want stable employer customers.

The trap isn't incidental—it's the primary function. Healthcare dependency keeps workers employed. Employment coercion maintains corporate workforces. The system is working exactly as those who benefit from it intend.

Entrepreneurs trapped by healthcare costs, workers locked into bad jobs by health insurance, talented people whose business ideas die because they can't afford individual coverage—these aren't system failures. They're the system working as designed. The design serves employer interests by limiting worker mobility and preventing entrepreneurship that would compete with established corporations.

This is healthcare as employment handcuffs. Healthcare as an entrepreneurship barrier. Healthcare as mechanism for maintaining corporate power over workers who should have the freedom to leave jobs that don't serve them, start businesses based on their skills, and pursue opportunities without risking their families' access to medical care.

Every other developed country has recognized that tying healthcare to employment is economically inefficient and unjust. They've separated healthcare from employment status, enabling entrepreneurship and labor mobility while ensuring everyone has healthcare access regardless of how they earn income.

The United States maintains employer-based insurance not because it's the best system but because it serves employer interests. We sacrifice entrepreneurship, innovation, labor mobility, and economic freedom to preserve a system that gives corporations power over workers by controlling access to healthcare.

The trap is deliberate. The harm is intentional. The system is working exactly as those who benefit from it designed it to work, and it will continue working this way—trapping workers, preventing entrepreneurship, stifling innovation, maintaining corporate power—until we choose to design a better system that separates healthcare from employment and makes healthcare access a right rather than a privilege contingent on maintaining corporate employment.

> *Systems built on cruelty can only suppress rage for so long. Eventually, the pressure finds a release. On December 4, 2024, it finally did.*

Research Notes:

This chapter integrates economic research on "job lock," entrepreneurship barriers created by employer-based insurance, and international comparisons showing higher entrepreneurship rates in countries with universal healthcare. The core arguments are based on documented economic effects of tying healthcare to employment, the deliberate misclassification of gig workers to avoid providing healthcare, and the structural mechanisms that benefit employers while harming workers and economic dynamism.

PART 3

THE RESISTANCE

CHAPTER 8

When The CEO Fell

December 4, 2024 - 6:45 AM

Brian Thompson walked out of the New York Hilton Midtown at 6:44 in the morning on December 4, 2024. He was heading to UnitedHealthcare's investor conference—an event where he would present the company's financial performance to the people who profited from his leadership. He never made it inside.

A man had been waiting for him. Not randomly positioned, not there by accident. Waiting specifically for Thompson, CEO of UnitedHealthcare, the largest health insurance company in America. The shooter knew his schedule. Knew his route. Knew exactly when he'd emerge from the hotel on West 54th Street in Midtown Manhattan.

Three shots at close range. Thompson fell. The shooter fled on foot, then switched to an electric bicycle, disappearing toward Central Park. The NYPD would later confirm what was obvious from the execution: this was targeted, deliberate, planned. This wasn't random violence. This was an assassination.

On the shell casings left at the scene, investigators found three words: "Delay." "Deny." "Depose."

Not random words. Not meaningless. These were the words describing the strategy that insurance companies use to avoid paying for healthcare: delay claims processing hoping people give up, deny coverage initially as standard practice, and depose—drag out legal challenges until people die or go bankrupt. The words came from a book documenting insurance industry practices, turned into a manifesto etched on bullets.

Brian Thompson, 50 years old, CEO since 2021, earning $10.2 million annually overseeing a company with $400 billion in revenue, died on a Manhattan sidewalk because someone decided to send a message about American healthcare using the language insurance companies use every day: deny, defend, depose.

The nation's attention turned immediately to New York. A CEO assassinated in broad daylight in Manhattan. A targeted killing. A manhunt. This should have generated the predictable response: shock, horror, condemnation, mourning.

That's not what happened.

What We Expected vs. What Happened

When a CEO is murdered, America has a script. The media expresses shock. Colleagues issue statements about a dedicated leader taken too soon. The public offers condolences. Politicians condemn violence. The story focuses on the tragedy of a life cut short, a family left grieving, the dangerous precedent of targeting business leaders.

Brian Thompson's murder broke the script completely.

Within hours, social media exploded—not with sympathy but with memes. Not with mourning but with dark humor. Not with condemnation but with something between understanding and celebration.

The jokes came fast.

They were brutal, and widespread.

They weren't fringe responses from isolated trolls.

They were mainstream.

Millions of Americans saw the news that a health insurance CEO had been assassinated and their immediate reaction was to make jokes about insurance denials.

Wanted posters appeared with faces of other healthcare executives—not threats exactly, but something that looked like accountability lists. Who profits from denying us care? Here are their names and faces.

Luigi Mangione, the alleged shooter who was arrested five days later in Altoona, Pennsylvania, developed instant fan clubs. A 26-year-old Ivy League educated man from a wealthy Maryland family became a folk hero for allegedly killing a health insurance executive.

The media was horrified. How could people react this way? Where was the empathy? Why weren't Americans mourning a man who'd been murdered in cold blood on a city street?

The answer was simple, and millions of Americans understood it instinctively: because we know exactly what UnitedHealthcare does. We know what Brian Thompson oversaw. We know the harm his company inflicts daily. Most of all, we're done pretending that harm is acceptable just because it's legal and profitable.

This wasn't ignorance or cruelty from the public. It was recognition. Americans recognized that the violence committed against Brian Thompson on December 4th was one man's death. The violence UnitedHealthcare commits is systematic, widespread, ongoing, and kills far more people—it just does it quietly, one denied claim at a time, without dramatic headlines or shell casings bearing messages.

The public response wasn't celebrating murder. It was recognizing reciprocal cruelty. You deny us healthcare, we deny you sympathy. The transaction was complete.

Who Was Brian Thompson?

Brian Thompson became CEO of UnitedHealthcare in April 2021. He'd worked for UnitedHealth Group since 2004, rising through the ranks during the company's massive expansion into Medicare Advantage and its increasing use of aggressive utilization management—industry speak for finding ways to deny coverage.

By 2024, UnitedHealthcare was the largest health insurer in America, part of UnitedHealth Group with $400.3 billion in revenue and $32.3 billion in operating earnings. Thompson earned $10.2 million in 2023—a compensation package that included base salary, performance-based incentives, and stock awards tied to the company's financial performance.

His performance was measured by profit. The company's profit came from premiums collected minus claims paid. The more claims denied, the higher the profit. The higher the profit, the larger Thompson's compensation. His financial incentives were directly tied to preventing people from accessing healthcare they'd paid for.

Under Thompson's leadership, UnitedHealthcare became known for aggressive denial practices. The company publicly stated it paid or approved approximately 90% of claims shortly after submission—a number that sounds good until you understand that the remaining 10% often included the most expensive, most necessary, most life-saving care. Routine claims got paid. Cancer treatment, experimental therapies, expensive medications, long-term care—these faced "additional review," which often meant denial.

The denial rates were documented. Medicare Advantage prior authorization data from 2023 showed that across the industry, 49.8 million prior authorization requests resulted in 6.4% being fully or partially denied. That sounds like a small percentage until you calculate that 6.4% of 49.8 million is over 3 million denials. Three million times someone needed care, their doctor said they needed it, and insurance said no.

For UnitedHealthcare specifically, post-acute care denial rates told an even starker story. A U.S. Senate Permanent Subcommittee on Investigations staff report documented that UnitedHealthcare's denial rates for post-acute care—the rehabilitation and skilled nursing care people need after hospitalizations—increased dramatically during Thompson's tenure: 10.9% in 2020, 16.3% in 2021, 22.7% in 2022. The denials more than doubled in two years. The Senate report noted this increase coincided with increased use of automated decision systems—AI algorithms designed to deny care faster and more efficiently than human reviewers.

Thompson oversaw the implementation of these systems. He knew denial rates were increasing. He knew automation was being used to reject care. He knew people were being denied coverage for medically necessary treatment. He knew because the Senate was investigating it, because advocacy groups were documenting it, because patients and providers were screaming about it.

He kept doing it because it was profitable.

The Department of Justice was investigating UnitedHealth Group for Medicare Advantage billing practices—specifically, for allegedly inflating patient diagnoses to receive higher government payments while simultaneously denying care to those same patients. Criminal and civil investigations were active. Reuters and the Wall Street Journal reported the DOJ's inquiries into systematic fraud. Thompson's company was under federal investigation for potentially defrauding the government and patients simultaneously.

He kept collecting his $10 million annual compensation.

Brian Thompson wasn't just a CEO. He was the architect of a denial system that impacted millions of Americans. Every prior authorization that took weeks while a patient's condition worsened. Every claim denied for "medical necessity" despite a doctor saying treatment was necessary. Every family that went bankrupt paying out-of-pocket for care insurance refused to cover. Every person who died waiting for approval that never came.

Thompson wasn't personally reviewing each denial. He didn't personally input the algorithms. But he oversaw the system, and he profited from it. He implemented the automation that increased denials. He bore responsibility for the harm his company inflicted systematically and deliberately.

The wealth he accumulated—the $10 million annually, the stock awards, the performance bonuses—was built on preventing people from accessing healthcare. Every dollar of profit his company made was a dollar collected in premiums but not paid out for care. His compensation increased when more claims were denied. His success required other people's suffering.

He knew. He absolutely knew. He still did it anyway because it was extraordinarily profitable.

"Delay, Deny, Depose"

The words on the shell casings referenced "Delay, Deny, Defend"—the title of a book by law professor Jay Feinman documenting how insurance companies systematically avoid paying legitimate claims. The book, published in 2010, laid out the three-part strategy:

Delay claims processing. Make it take weeks or months for routine approvals. Create bureaucratic barriers. Require repeated submissions of the same documentation. Transfer calls between departments. Put people on hold. Make accessing coverage so difficult and time-consuming that some percentage of people give up before getting care. Each day of delay is a day the insurance company keeps the premium payment without providing the coverage.

Deny claims initially as standard practice. The first answer is always no. Deny for "lack of medical necessity" even when doctors say treatment is necessary. Deny for "experimental" when treatments are FDA-approved. Deny for "not covered under your plan" and hope people don't appeal. Deny and force patients to fight for coverage they already paid for. A significant percentage won't appeal. Those denials become pure profit—premiums collected, no care provided.

Defend denials when challenged. Create appeal processes that require multiple levels of review. Demand extensive documentation. Use medical review companies staffed by doctors who've never seen the patient to overrule treating physicians. Drag out appeals for months. Make the process so exhausting that people give up. If they still persist, deploy legal teams to defend the denial in court if necessary. Make fighting the denial more expensive and time-consuming than paying out-of-pocket.

The book added a fourth D that the shooter modified to "Depose": use legal processes to delay until the problem resolves itself—meaning the patient dies, gives up, or goes bankrupt. Draw out litigation. File motions. Demand depositions. Make the legal process so costly and slow that winning becomes impossible for individual patients fighting multi-billion dollar corporations.

This strategy isn't some conspiracy theory. It's documented industry practice. Insurance companies don't hide it, they call it "utilization management" and "cost containment." They present it as responsible stewardship of healthcare dollars. They frame it as preventing fraud and unnecessary care.

What patients experience, though, is deny, delay, defend—systematic barriers to accessing care they paid for. Bureaucratic cruelty designed to prevent treatment. A system where the first answer is always no and getting to yes requires fighting the company you're paying to provide coverage.

The shooter knew this playbook. He knew it so well he etched it on bullets. Three words—delay, deny, depose—that summarized exactly how Brian Thompson's company operated. How it made $32 billion in operating earnings while denying coverage to people dying from cancer, recovering from strokes, needing post-hospitalization rehabilitation.

The American public recognized those words immediately. They didn't need the reference explained. They knew "delay, deny, defend" because they'd lived it. Every person who'd fought with insurance over prior authorization knew. Every family bankrupted by denied claims knew. Every person who'd died waiting for coverage approval knew, or their families knew.

The shell casings were a diagnosis, not just a message. They named the disease, and millions of Americans who saw those words understood exactly what they meant because they'd been subjected to that system themselves.

The Memes: Dark Humor as Truth-Telling

Within hours of Thompson's death, social media transformed into a collective dark comedy show.

The memes were devastatingly on point.

"Prior authorization required for sympathy—please submit thoughts and prayers form in triplicate and allow 6-8 weeks for processing."

"Unfortunately, this CEO was out-of-network. You'll be responsible for the full cost of grieving."

"Claim denied: condolences not medically necessary."

"Have you tried Tylenol and rest before seeking sympathy for a gunshot wound?"

"Your request for empathy has been denied. You may appeal this decision by submitting documentation from three independent witnesses proving you deserved to live."

The jokes weren't isolated. They were everywhere— Reddit, Facebook, TikTok, and Instagram. Millions of Americans participated. They shared their own insurance horror stories alongside the jokes. They posted denial letters. They documented prior authorization nightmares. They calculated how much they'd paid in premiums versus how much their insurance actually covered.

Healthcare workers—nurses, doctors, medical assistants, administrators—posted about fighting insurance companies on behalf of patients. They described spending hours on peer-to-peer review calls trying to convince insurance company doctors to approve care that treating physicians said was necessary; watching patients deteriorate while waiting for authorization that took weeks; delivering news that coverage was denied for treatment that could save someone's life.

The memes weren't coming from people who didn't understand healthcare. They were coming from people who understood it intimately—as patients, as family members of patients, as healthcare workers trapped in a system designed to deny care while extracting profit.

Luigi Mangione merchandise appeared within days. T-shirts, hats, and mugs, all celebrating the alleged shooter. "Free Luigi" became a rallying cry. Social media accounts dedicated to supporting him gained hundreds of thousands of followers. Young people especially (18-29 year-olds according to polling) saw him as something between folk hero and revolutionary. Someone who finally made a healthcare executive pay a price for the suffering the industry inflicts.

The media—as I said earlier—was horrified. How could people celebrate a murderer? Where was the empathy? Where was the humanity? What kind of society jokes about assassination?

What the media missed was what the memes were actually doing. They weren't celebrating murder. They were processing trauma through humor. They were expressing rage that had been building for decades with nowhere to go. They were engaging in collective truth-telling: the insurance industry kills people for profit, and we're done pretending that's acceptable just because it's legal.

Humor is how traumatized people cope. Dark humor especially. When you can't change the situation, when you're powerless against a system designed to harm you, when speaking plainly gets you labeled as unreasonable or radical, you joke. You make memes. You use irony and sarcasm to say what you can't say directly.

The memes said clearly: Brian Thompson profited from denying us healthcare. He got rich while we went bankrupt. He lived in luxury while people died from denied coverage. Now he's dead, and we're supposed to mourn? We're supposed to pretend his death is a tragedy greater than the thousands who died from denials he oversaw?

No. We're done pretending.

The jokes weren't lack of empathy. They were reciprocal treatment. Insurance companies show no empathy when they deny cancer treatment. They show no empathy when they bankrupt families. They show no empathy when people die waiting for authorization. They've taught Americans exactly how much empathy to show when insurance executives face consequences: none.

The memes were a collective recognition: this man represented a system designed to harm us. He profited from our suffering. He made millions while we fought for coverage we'd paid for. When someone finally made him pay a price, we weren't sad. We were relieved that for once, the person inflicting harm faced consequences instead of receiving bonuses.

The transaction was complete. You deny us healthcare, we deny you sympathy.

Where was the empathy when insurance denials killed people? Where was the empathy when cancer patients died waiting for prior authorization? Where was the empathy when families lost their homes to medical debt? Where was the empathy when people with chronic conditions went bankrupt paying out-of-pocket for care insurance refused to cover?

There was none. Insurance companies operate without empathy because empathy doesn't generate profit. They've systematically removed empathy from healthcare, replacing it with algorithms designed to maximize denial rates and minimize payouts.

So Americans responded with the same lack of empathy. The memes weren't cruel. They were mirroring exactly what insurance companies do daily. The cruelty was reciprocal, and millions of Americans participated because they recognized the truth: Brian Thompson's death was one man. Insurance company policies kill thousands annually. Which deserves more grief?

What the Public Response Revealed

The collective response to a healthcare CEO's assassination wasn't fringe. It wasn't limited to extremist corners of the internet. It was mainstream, and it revealed something critical about American healthcare: people know.

They *know* the system is designed to harm them. They *know* insurance companies profit from denying care. They *know* executives get rich while patients die. And they're done pretending any of this is acceptable.

National polling documented the response. A NORC/Associated Press poll conducted December 12-16, 2024, just days after the shooting, found that while a majority assigned primary responsibility for the killing to the shooter himself, significant percentages also cited insurance company profits and coverage denials as contributing factors. Americans weren't justifying murder, but they were diagnosing the conditions that made someone desperate enough to commit it.

An Emerson College poll from December 2024 found that while an overall majority found the killing unacceptable, there was stark age-based divergence. Younger respondents—18-29 year-olds—showed significantly different response patterns than older Americans. They were more likely to understand why it happened, less likely to unconditionally condemn it, more likely to see it as a consequence of systemic failure rather than isolated violence.

An Economist/YouGov poll measured favorability ratings toward Luigi Mangione, the alleged shooter. That such a poll existed at all—measuring public favorability toward an accused murderer—demonstrated how far outside normal bounds the public response had fallen.

The generational variation in responses showed that younger Americans, who've grown up entirely within the for-profit healthcare system and face decades more of fighting insurance companies, saw Mangione very differently than their parents' generation.

These weren't fringe opinions. These were mainstream responses captured by major polling organizations. Millions of Americans looked at a CEO assassination and said: I understand why this happened. I don't necessarily condone it, but I understand it. The system creates this rage. The cruelty is systemic and deliberate. Someone finally made them pay.

The public response revealed that Americans have been paying attention. They know insurance companies systematically deny care. They know executives earn millions while patients go bankrupt. They know the profit motive kills people. They know prior authorization is designed to delay and deny. They know algorithms are deployed to reject claims faster than humans could. They know the entire system is structured to collect premiums while minimizing coverage.

They know because they've experienced it. Every family has healthcare horror stories. Denied claims. Surprise bills. Prior authorization nightmares. Medical debt. Fighting for coverage they'd paid for. Watching family members deteriorate while insurance companies dragged out authorization. Going bankrupt despite having insurance. Choosing between medications and groceries because insurance wouldn't cover prescriptions.

The collective knowledge is comprehensive. Americans understand the system intimately because they live inside it. They're not confused about why healthcare costs so much and covers so little. They're not mystified by high premiums and high deductibles. They know exactly where the money goes: to insurance company profits and executive compensation.

Brian Thompson's $10.2 million annual salary came from somewhere. It came from premiums collected but not paid out for care. It came from denied claims. It came from prior authorizations that took so long people gave up or died waiting. It came from the systematic extraction of profit from suffering.

Americans *know* this. The public response to his death revealed collective understanding that healthcare executives aren't healers or administrators serving the public good—they're profiteers extracting wealth from a captive population that needs medical care to survive. They profit from denying care. Their wealth is built on other people's suffering. Their success requires people to die from preventable conditions or go bankrupt paying for treatment out-of-pocket.

When millions of Americans implicitly understand the motives behind a CEO's assassination, the problem isn't the millions of Americans. The problem is what the CEO represented and enacted. The problem is a system so cruel, so predatory, so deliberately harmful that people who would never normally condone violence look at a healthcare executive's murder and think: he had it coming.

That response—widespread, mainstream, persistent—is a diagnosis. It's not a diagnosis of American bloodthirstiness or moral decay. It's a diagnosis of systemic failure so profound that people can't muster sympathy when architects of that system face consequences.

Americans aren't confused about who's harming them. They know, and they always have. Thompson's assassination just revealed how widespread that knowledge is, and how exhausted Americans are with pretending the system serves them rather than exploiting them.

"Deny, Defend, Depose"—NOT Justifying Violence

This chapter must be explicit about something: Brian Thompson's murder was wrong. Killing him didn't fix healthcare. It didn't change insurance company practices. It didn't save anyone from denied coverage. Violence isn't the solution to systemic problems. Luigi Mangione, if guilty, committed murder and will face legal consequences as he should.

Condemning the murder is not the same as defending the system that motivated it.

Understanding the rage that produced the killing is not the same as endorsing the killing.

Refusing to mourn Brian Thompson is not the same as celebrating his death.

These distinctions matter. The response to his assassination has been deliberately conflated: if you understand why someone would kill a healthcare CEO, you must support murder. If you won't mourn him, you must be pro-violence. If you acknowledge the harm insurance companies inflict, you must justify assassinating their executives.

This is false logic designed to shut down conversation about systemic harm by making any acknowledgment of that harm appear to justify violence.

The truth is more complex: Thompson's killing was wrong, and the system he oversaw kills far more people through legal means. One murder doesn't justify another, but comparing one assassination to systematic denial of care that kills thousands annually—bankrupting hundreds of thousands more—reveals which violence is actually greater.

Thompson died from gunshot wounds on a Manhattan sidewalk. That's violence. It's visible, dramatic, immediate. One man, one killer, one death. The violence is obvious and undeniable.

Insurance companies kill people through denied coverage. People die from cancer that could have been treated if chemotherapy hadn't been denied as "not medically necessary." People die from heart attacks that could have been prevented if cardiac medications hadn't been denied as "not covered under your plan." People die from infections that could have been stopped if antibiotics hadn't been denied pending "additional review."

These deaths are quieter. They don't happen on city sidewalks in front of witnesses. They happen in hospitals where dying patients are told insurance won't cover the treatment that could save them. They happen at home, where people ration medications because insurance won't cover adequate doses. They happen slowly, over weeks and months of denied appeals and delayed authorizations, until the patient is too sick to save.

The insurance company violence is systematic, widespread, ongoing, and legal. It kills more people than isolated assassinations ever could—but it's not dramatic. It doesn't generate headlines. It doesn't have shell casings bearing messages. It's just spreadsheets showing denied claims and quarterly earnings reports showing record profits.

Which is the greater violence?

Thompson's death: one man, murdered, undeniably tragic for his family and people who knew him personally.

Insurance denial deaths: thousands annually, dying from preventable conditions because coverage was denied, equally tragic for their families but lacking dramatic headlines or national attention.

Medical bankruptcies: 530,000 families annually destroyed financially despite having health insurance, their lives derailed by debts they'll never pay off, many ultimately losing homes and savings to pay for care insurance refused to cover.

Which represents more harm? Which causes more suffering? Which destroys more lives?

The answer is obvious. This doesn't justify Thompson's murder. It contextualizes the public response to his death.

Americans weren't celebrating murder. They were recognizing proportionality. The media demanded grief for one CEO. The public responded: where's the grief for thousands killed by insurance denials? Where's the outrage at systematic harm? Where's the accountability for executives who profit from suffering?

The public refused to participate in mourning theater that pretended Thompson's death was uniquely tragic while ignoring the tragedy his company inflicted daily. That refusal wasn't pro-violence. It was pro-honesty. It was insisting on acknowledging the full scope of violence, not just the illegal kind that generates headlines.

This is what the media couldn't understand: Americans weren't confused about right and wrong. They understood perfectly that murder is wrong. They also understood that systematic denial of healthcare is wrong. They refused to pretend only one of these things mattered while ignoring the other.

Condemning Thompson's murder while defending the insurance industry's systematic harm is moral incoherence. Both are wrong. Both cause suffering. Both kill people. One is illegal; the other is profitable. That's the only difference.

The public response said clearly: we understand both forms of violence. We condemn both. But we won't mourn the architect of systematic harm while ignoring the victims of that harm. We won't pretend one CEO's death is more tragic than thousands of deaths from denied coverage. We won't participate in grief theater that centers executives while erasing patients.

As stated, this isn't justifying violence. It's demanding consistent moral standards. If Thompson's death is tragic—and it is—then so are the deaths caused by policies he oversaw. If killing one person is wrong—and it is—then systematic denial of healthcare that kills thousands is also wrong. If Mangione should face consequences for murder—and he should—then executives whose policies kill people should face consequences too.

The difference is that Mangione will go to prison. Thompson died, but the insurance company policies continue. The denials continue, the bankruptcies continue, the deaths continue, and the executives who oversee these systems continue collecting multimillion-dollar compensation packages with no legal consequences, no public accountability, no threat to their wealth or freedom.

Americans understand this asymmetry. They understand that violence is punished only when it's illegal, not when it's profitable. They understand that killing one CEO gets you arrested while systematic policies that kill thousands get you bonuses and promotions.

That understanding—widespread, mainstream, undeniable—explains the public response to Thompson's death. It's a clear-eyed recognition that the system punishes individual violence while rewarding systematic violence, and that this asymmetry is itself unjust.

Understanding the Rage as Rational

I was sitting in my car on my lunch break, scrolling through YouTube, when I found out Brian Thompson had been shot. I saw the headline and knew immediately why he'd been killed.

Not because I'm psychic. Not because I knew anything about Luigi Mangione or his motivations. I knew because I work in this system. I know what insurance companies do. I know how UnitedHealthcare operates. I knew that somewhere, someone had been pushed past the breaking point by denied coverage, bankrupted by medical bills, traumatized by watching a family member die from preventable causes because insurance wouldn't pay for treatment.

I felt nothing. No shock. No sympathy. No horror. Just recognition: something like this was bound to happen. It finally did. Maybe now healthcare will be taken seriously in this country.

I went back to work. My coworkers were shocked. They speculated that maybe Thompson was having an affair and that's what triggered the murder—some personal vendetta, a jealous spouse, a private matter. They were curious about the mystery, eager to know more details.

I wasn't. I knew deep down that the shooter felt oppressed by the healthcare system. I knew that was the reason before any details came out. I stayed silent. My colleagues were shocked. I understood completely. Our reactions couldn't have been more different.

Days later, when the details emerged—the shell casings, the alleged manifesto, the targeting of a healthcare CEO specifically—my colleagues were surprised. I wasn't. Of course it was about healthcare. Of course it was about insurance denials. Of course someone finally decided that if the system won't hold executives accountable, maybe individuals will.

When Luigi Mangione was arrested, the media narrative was simple: a deranged killer caught, justice served, case closed.

But that's not what I saw happening outside the news cycle. I saw millions of Americans expressing something darker—not celebration of violence, but recognition. Understanding. A grim sense that this was inevitable.

I don't condone what happened. Violence isn't the answer. But I do understand the rage that made millions of people see a CEO's murder and think: Finally, someone who profits from this system faced a consequence."

I've watched patients suffer from denied coverage. I've fought insurance companies for prior authorizations while patients deteriorated waiting for approval. I've told patients that insurance won't cover treatment and watched families calculate whether they can afford to pay out-of-pocket or whether they'll just have to go without care they need.

I pay too much for healthcare myself. I hate the system for myself and for my patients. Healthcare is profit-driven in the United States and it shouldn't be. We pay premiums, then we pay deductibles, then we pay coinsurance, then we get surprise bills for things we thought were covered. We spend an exorbitant amount of money for insurance premiums, then more for deductibles and out-of-pocket maximums.

I'm a healthcare provider. When I pick up locums shifts, I make good money. I can afford marketplace coverage even though it's expensive and unstable. Imagine what it's like for people earning poverty wages, for people with chronic conditions, for families with children who need ongoing care. Imagine being trapped between paying rent and paying for medications. Imagine watching a family member die because treatment was denied as "not medically necessary" despite doctors saying it was the only chance for survival.

That's the rage. That's what produces someone desperate enough to wait on a Manhattan sidewalk at 6:44 in the morning and shoot a healthcare CEO three times. Not mental illness. Not irrationality. Rage at a system designed to harm people for profit; at executives who get rich from that harm; at the complete absence of accountability for legal violence that kills thousands while illegal violence that kills one gets national headlines and a manhunt.

The rage is rational. It's appropriate. It's the predictable result of decades of systematic cruelty inflicted by a healthcare system designed to extract profit while denying care.

Americans have been harmed by this system for their entire lives. Every family has stories. Denied claims. Medical bankruptcies. Loved ones who died from preventable conditions because insurance wouldn't cover treatment. The harm is universal, widespread, and deliberate.

When a system deliberately harms people, rage is rational. When executives profit from that harm, directing rage at those executives is rational. When legal accountability doesn't exist, people seeking other forms of accountability is predictable if not justifiable.

Thompson's assassination made it visible that insurance companies kill people quietly, one denial at a time.

Thompson's death was spectacular, which is why it got attention, but the daily deaths from insurance denials are equally real. They just don't make headlines.

The public response diagnosed this reality.

The rage isn't irrational. When you inflict harm systematically, deliberately, for profit, for decades, people eventually respond with rage. That's not mysterious. That's predictable. That's human nature.

The mystery isn't the motive behind Thompson's murder. The mystery is why it didn't happen sooner. The mystery is how insurance executives have operated with complete impunity for so long, profiting from harm while facing no consequences, no accountability, no threat to their wealth or safety.

Thompson's death ended that impunity for one executive. It revealed that accountability can come from unexpected directions when legal accountability doesn't exist. It demonstrated that executives who profit from harm are not invulnerable, not untouchable, not immune to consequences just because their violence is legal.

Millions of Americans looked at that revelation and felt something between relief and satisfaction. Not because they're pro-murder, but because finally, for once, someone who inflicted systematic harm faced consequences instead of receiving bonuses.

That response is rational, and appropriate. It's the predictable result of a system that punishes only illegal violence while rewarding legal violence that causes vastly more harm.

What This Revealed About American Healthcare

The assassination of a healthcare CEO was a symptom, not a cause. The disease is the system itself.

When millions of Americans celebrate or understand a CEO's murder, the CEO isn't the problem. The system that made his actions profitable is the problem. The system that rewarded him for denying care is the problem. The system that gave him $10 million annually while patients went bankrupt is the problem.

Thompson was one executive. Replace him and the system continues unchanged. Deny, delay, defend are company policies, not individual decisions. Automated denial algorithms continue running regardless of who's CEO. Prior authorization requirements remain regardless of who oversees them. The profit motive that makes denial financially rewarding persists regardless of individual executives.

This is what Americans understand instinctively when they refuse to mourn Thompson. They understand that he represented a system, not just himself. Killing him didn't fix that system. It revealed how broken the system is—so broken that people couldn't muster sympathy when one architect of systematic harm faced consequences.

The public response revealed collective understanding that extends far beyond Thompson's death, and points to the truth about the system I have laid out this far:

Insurance companies are predatory. They profit from denying care, not providing it. Their business model depends on collecting premiums while minimizing payouts. Every dollar not spent on patient care is a dollar of profit. The financial incentives are completely misaligned with healthcare outcomes. Keeping people healthy doesn't generate profit. Denying coverage for expensive treatments does.

The system is designed to extract profit while denying care. It's not broken. It's working exactly as designed. High premiums, high deductibles, narrow networks, prior authorization requirements, automated denial systems, byzantine appeals processes—all of these are features, not bugs. They're designed to make accessing care difficult enough that some percentage of people give up before getting coverage they paid for.

Executives get rich while patients die. This particular CEO earned $10.2 million. Patients went bankrupt. This isn't a coincidence or an unfortunate side effect. It's the system working as designed: extract maximum value from patients through premiums, deny maximum care through utilization management, and transfer the resulting profit to executives and shareholders.

There's no accountability for legal harm. Insurance companies can deny coverage that results in deaths and face no consequences beyond occasional regulatory fines that amount to tiny fractions of annual profits. Executives whose policies kill people face no legal penalties, no threat to their wealth or freedom, no personal accountability for systematic harm. The violence they oversee is legal, therefore it's acceptable, therefore it continues.

Americans are not confused about how healthcare works or why it's so expensive and inadequate. They know exactly what's happening: they're being exploited by a for-profit system designed to extract maximum revenue while providing minimum care.

Thompson's assassination only crystallized this understanding. For one moment, the usual justifications and euphemisms didn't work. You couldn't pretend insurance companies were benign, that denials were rare mistakes, or the system served patients rather than shareholders. You couldn't pretend executives bore no responsibility for the harm their companies inflicted systematically.

The public response forced honesty. Americans hate the healthcare system. They hate it because it harms them deliberately. They hate it because executives get rich from their suffering. So when one of those executives died, they didn't mourn—because he represented everything that's killing them.

This isn't about one CEO. It's about every denied claim, every bankrupted family, every preventable death, every prior authorization nightmare, every person who died waiting for insurance approval, every patient who rationed medications because insurance wouldn't cover adequate doses, every family destroyed by medical debt despite having insurance.

Thompson represented all of it by leading a company that denied coverage systematically, automated denial, and increased denial rates, all while decreasing time spent reviewing individual cases. His compensation increased when denials increased. His success required patient suffering.

Americans understood that demanding sympathy for a CEO who showed no sympathy when denying life-saving care was asking them to participate in a lie.

They refused. The refusal revealed that Americans understand that the system is sick by design. They know the cruelty is intentional. They know the profit motive kills people. They know executives bear responsibility for that harm.

Thompson's death made that knowledge visible and undeniable. For once, Americans could say plainly what they usually have to whisper or express through dark humor: the people running this system are killing us for profit, and we're done pretending that's acceptable.

The Moment I Knew This Book Had to Be Written

I realized sitting in my car that lunch break that the U.S. needs to get with the program. Our healthcare system sucks for both patients and providers. We—patients—go broke paying for monthly insurance premiums, then broke again covering deductibles and balanced billing. Then we do it all over again on January 1st when everything resets and gets even more expensive.

And providers? We're trained in preventive medicine, but the system doesn't give us time to practice it or prioritize it. Fifteen-minute appointments, endless documentation, and exhaustion wear us down until we stop fighting. We become complicit—treating illness instead of preventing it, participating in a system designed to harm the people we're supposed to help.

Thompson's assassination revealed that Americans are ready to hear what I've been seeing for years: the system is designed this way. The harm is intentional, the cruelty serves profit, and the people running this system are responsible for what it does.

This book exists because that fury needs diagnosis. Americans are right to be enraged. The system is designed to harm them. The cruelty is intentional. The profit motive does kill people. Thompson's death revealed what millions already knew, and now we can say it plainly without being dismissed as radical or extreme.

The system is sick by design. Not broken—but designed this way. Not failing—but succeeding at its actual purpose of extracting profit while denying care. Not needing reform—but needing replacement.

This is why the book needed to be written now. Because the moment of clarity has arrived. Because Americans are ready to hear what they already know. Because the rage is rational and the system is indefensible. Someone needs to say plainly what the memes said in dark humor: the people running this system are killing us for profit, and we're done pretending that's acceptable.

Brian Thompson died December 4, 2024. The American healthcare system has been killing people systematically for decades. One death made headlines. The other continues quietly, profitably, legally.

This book is about the ongoing violence, not the spectacular exception. It's about the system designed to harm, not the individual who finally snapped. It's about the cruelty that's acceptable because it's profitable, not the cruelty that's condemned because it's illegal.

Thompson's assassination revealed that Americans understand the difference. They know which violence is greater. They know who bears responsibility, and they're ready to demand accountability for systematic harm that dwarfs any individual act of violence.

The rage is rational. The fury is justified. The system is sick by design.

Now, finally, we can say so plainly.

> *The system bankrupts even the insured. But at least now, insurance companies can't use your medical history as a weapon to deny you coverage entirely. The Affordable Care Act is imperfect. Whether you love the ACA or hate it, you're protected by it.*

Research Notes:

This chapter synthesizes verified reporting from Reuters, Associated Press, Wall Street Journal, U.S. Senate Permanent Subcommittee on Investigations reports, Kaiser Family Foundation data, and national polling from NORC, Emerson College, and Economist/YouGov. The documented public response, denial rate data, and Thompson's compensation are from public records and mainstream media reporting. The personal perspective reflects the author's experience as a healthcare provider witnessing both the shooting's aftermath and the systemic harm insurance companies inflict daily.

CHAPTER

9 The ACA Under Siege

The Woman Who Lost Her Coverage

The following scenario is a composite constructed from patterns documented during Medicaid unwinding. The details are hypothetical, but the dynamics are real and widespread.

Maria Rodriguez had finally felt secure. After years of working part-time jobs without benefits, Texas expanded Medicaid in 2023, and she qualified for coverage. For the first time in her adult life, she could see a doctor without calculating whether she could afford it. Her diabetes medications were covered. Her blood pressure was under control. She felt, for the first time in years, like her health wasn't a crisis waiting to happen.

Then the political winds shifted. The state threatened to add work requirements to Medicaid. Maria worked sixteen hours per week at a retail job—all her chronic conditions allowed her to manage—but the new requirements demanded thirty hours of documented work activity plus monthly paperwork proving compliance. She tried to increase her hours, but her employer wouldn't give her full-time work (full-time employees cost more in benefits). She tried to document her hours properly, but the forms were complex and the deadlines unforgiving.

She missed a deadline. Not because she wasn't working. Not because she was lazy or trying to cheat the system. She missed it because she was working, taking care of her mother, managing her own health conditions, and trying to navigate bureaucratic requirements designed to be difficult to meet.

Her coverage was terminated.

Within three months, she couldn't afford her diabetes medications. Her blood sugar spiraled out of control. She ended up in the emergency room with diabetic ketoacidosis—a completely preventable crisis that cost the system thousands of dollars and nearly killed her. The ER stabilized her and discharged her with prescriptions she couldn't afford to fill. She'd had insurance. The state took it away. Now she was back where she started: sick, scared, and one medical emergency away from financial catastrophe.

This is what "Medicaid reform" actually means. This is what happens when states add punitive requirements designed not to encourage work but to kick people off coverage. This is the reality of fighting for scraps of dignity in a system designed to exclude the people who need help most.

What the ACA Actually Did

Before we talk about what's under attack, we need to remember what the Affordable Care Act actually accomplished—because Americans, dangerously, have already started forgetting how bad things were before 2014.

The ACA eliminated pre-existing condition exclusions. Read that again and let it sink in, because this protection is so fundamental that it's easy to forget it didn't always exist. Before the ACA, if you'd ever had cancer, insurance companies could refuse to cover you. If you had diabetes, asthma, depression, or any of hundreds of other conditions, insurers could deny you coverage entirely or charge you premiums so high they were effectively denials.

I have pre-existing conditions that would have excluded me from insurance coverage before the ACA—or at minimum, would have raised my premiums significantly to the point where I couldn't afford coverage. This isn't unusual. Most everyone has a pre-existing condition: seasonal allergies, asthma, high blood pressure, PCOS, endometriosis, depression, anxiety, back pain. Among community health center patients who gained insurance post-ACA, over 70% had at least one pre-existing condition. The most common were mental health disorders, affecting 45.6% of those who gained Medicaid and 30.5% of those who gained private coverage.

Pre-existing condition protections aren't abstract policy—they're the difference between having access to healthcare and being permanently locked out of the insurance system because you got sick once.

The ACA allowed young adults to stay on their parents' insurance until age 26. By December 2011, 3.1 million young adults had gained coverage through this provision. Before the ACA, turning 18 or graduating college often meant losing health coverage at exactly the age when young people are establishing independence, starting careers, and least able to afford individual insurance.

The ACA required essential health benefits. Insurance plans had to cover hospitalization, emergency services, prescription drugs, mental health treatment, and maternity care. Before the ACA, many plans excluded maternity coverage entirely, forcing women to pay thousands out of pocket for prenatal care and delivery. Mental health coverage was optional, leaving people with depression, anxiety, and other treatable conditions unable to access care.

The ACA eliminated lifetime caps on coverage. Before 2014, many insurance plans set lifetime limits on how much they'd pay—often $1 million or $2 million. That sounds like a lot until your child is born premature and spends months in the NICU, or you're diagnosed with cancer requiring years of treatment. When you hit your lifetime cap, your insurance stopped paying. You were on your own for all future medical expenses. The ACA made this practice illegal.

The ACA eliminated gender-based premium ratings. Before 2014, insurance companies charged women higher premiums than men for the same coverage. Women paid more simply for being women—insurance companies justified this by pointing to maternity costs, as if pregnancy were a women-only decision and responsibility. The ACA made this discrimination illegal.

The ACA expanded Medicaid to cover all adults with incomes up to 138% of the federal poverty level. This single provision extended coverage to millions of low-income adults who'd previously had no access to affordable insurance. By 2022, Medicaid covered approximately 80.6 million people—24.2% of the U.S. population. The expansion was particularly impactful for racial and ethnic minorities: from 2010 to 2019, Medicaid coverage among low-income adults in expansion states increased by 11.2 percentage points for Black adults and 16.2 percentage points for Hispanic adults.

The ACA created health insurance marketplaces with income-based subsidies that made coverage affordable for middle-income people who didn't qualify for Medicaid and didn't have employer-sponsored insurance. As of 2024, more than 21 million people have signed up for marketplace coverage—up from 10.6 million in 2020.

The combined impact: the number of uninsured fell from 48.6 million (16% of the population) in 2010 to 28.6 million (9.1%) in 2015. Twenty million Americans gained health insurance. Of those, 13 million were insured through Medicaid.

These weren't radical reforms. These were basic human decency: don't deny coverage to sick people, don't kick people off insurance when they get expensive, don't charge women more than men, don't leave young adults uninsured, don't cap coverage at arbitrary limits that bankrupt families facing serious illness.

Americans have already started forgetting how cruel the pre-ACA insurance system was. That forgetting is dangerous, because what's being attacked right now are these fundamental protections that millions of people depend on for survival.

What the ACA Didn't Fix

The Affordable Care Act was an improvement. It helped millions of people. It's also inadequate, and understanding its limitations is essential to understanding both why it's under attack and why it's not the final solution American healthcare needs.

The ACA still leaves profit-driven insurance companies at the center of the healthcare system. It regulates those companies more strictly than before—they can't deny coverage for pre-existing conditions, can't impose lifetime caps, must cover essential benefits—but they're still for-profit entities whose business model depends on collecting premiums while minimizing payouts. The fundamental conflict of interest remains: insurance companies profit when they deny care.

Medical bankruptcy continues at catastrophic levels despite the ACA. As documented in Chapter 6, 62.1% of all bankruptcies are medical-related, affecting 530,000 families annually. Three-quarters of people filing medical bankruptcy had health insurance when they got sick. The ACA expanded coverage but didn't eliminate the high deductibles, coinsurance requirements, and out-of-pocket costs that bankrupt insured families.

The ACA didn't fix the reactive model. Insurance companies still profit more from treating illness than preventing it as discussed in Chapter 4. Fee-for-service payment still rewards volume over value. Primary care physicians still earn half what specialists make. Insurance churn still means companies don't benefit from investing in prevention. The ACA expanded who has coverage—it didn't change the incentive structure that prioritizes treatment over prevention.

Provider burnout and moral injury continue destroying the healthcare workforce despite the ACA. Between 48-53% of physicians are burned out, forced to fight insurance denials, spend more time on documentation than with patients, and participate in harmful cost-based rationing that violates their professional values—a crisis I examine in detail in Chapter 10. The ACA didn't address the conditions creating this workforce crisis.

Surprise billing continued until 2022—eight years after the ACA's main provisions took effect—and gaps in protection remain. Ground ambulances still aren't covered by the No Surprises Act. Patients still receive unexpected bills for care they couldn't avoid from providers they didn't choose.

Pharmaceutical price gouging remains completely unregulated under the ACA. Drug companies charge whatever they want. The United States pays far more for medications than any other developed nation, and the ACA did nothing to change this. Americans still ration insulin, skip doses of expensive medications, and choose between prescriptions and groceries because the ACA left pharmaceutical pricing untouched.

Since I work as a locums provider, I purchase my own insurance through the ACA marketplace. The coverage has been okay, but the cost is still outrageous with some plans. I've had to change insurance providers every couple of years either because of cost increases that made my plan unaffordable or because insurance carriers dropped coverage in my area entirely. This instability—having to switch insurers, lose access to established providers, start over with new networks—is built into the ACA marketplace system. It's better than having no coverage, but it's far from good healthcare.

The ACA was a significant improvement over what came before. It helped millions of people, including me. It's also fundamentally inadequate—a heavily compromised reform that preserved the profit-driven insurance system while adding regulations that insurance companies, hospitals, and pharmaceutical companies constantly work to undermine or circumvent.

Understanding both what the ACA accomplished and what it failed to fix is essential. It's worth defending against attacks that would eliminate even these inadequate protections. It's simultaneously insufficient as a final solution to American healthcare's structural cruelty. Both things are true. The ACA is simultaneously too important to lose and too limited to be where reform efforts end.

Medicaid Expansion Resistance: The Racist Geography of Refusal

The Affordable Care Act offered states a deal: expand Medicaid to cover all adults with incomes up to 138% of the federal poverty level, and the federal government would pay 100% of the costs for the first three years, then 90% permanently thereafter. This was an extraordinarily generous offer—states could extend health coverage to millions of their poorest residents at minimal state cost.

Then the Supreme Court made Medicaid expansion optional, and the racist geography of American healthcare policy revealed itself with brutal clarity.

As of 2024, ten states continue to reject Medicaid expansion. These states aren't randomly distributed across the country. They're concentrated in the South and align remarkably with states that fought hardest against civil rights, that resisted Medicare and Medicaid integration in the 1960s, and that have the highest percentages of Black residents.

The correlation isn't coincidence. It's continuation.

Medicaid was designed with racism built into its structure. When Medicare and Medicaid were created in 1965, President Lyndon B. Johnson cut a deal with Southern congressmen: Medicaid would be a joint federal-state program, giving states hostile to civil rights significant control over program benefits, funding, and the health of disproportionate numbers of Black beneficiaries. As Jamila Michener writes, "Medicaid is racialized, despite being facially colorblind, because race has been a central factor in shaping policies, discourse, design, implementation, and perceptions of it."

Medicaid expansion resistance continues this racist heritage. States with large Black populations would rather let poor people—disproportionately Black and Brown—die than expand coverage that would primarily benefit people of color. The cruelty isn't incidental. It's the point.

The human cost of this refusal is staggering. In the ten non-expansion states, individuals fall into a coverage gap: too poor to qualify for marketplace subsidies (which start at 100% of federal poverty level) but ineligible for Medicaid because their states refuse to expand. These are the working poor—people earning poverty wages at jobs that don't provide insurance, people too "rich" for restrictive state Medicaid programs but too poor to afford marketplace coverage even with subsidies.

They're trapped—deliberately—by state governments that chose ideology over their residents' lives.

From 2010 to 2019, Medicaid coverage among low-income adults in expansion states increased by 11.2 percentage points for Black adults and 16.2 percentage points for Hispanic adults. In non-expansion states, these gains didn't happen. Black and brown residents of non-expansion states watch people in neighboring expansion states access healthcare while they remain locked out—not because their states can't afford expansion (the federal government pays 90%), but because their states won't accept federal funding that would primarily benefit people of color.

Medicaid expansion since 2017 has covered at least 1.7 million additional people across seven states that expanded between 2017 and 2022, with millions more enrolling in North Carolina and South Dakota when they expanded in 2023. Every state that expands sees dramatic coverage gains. Every state that refuses sees people suffer and die preventably.

The federal government would pay 90% of expansion costs. States refusing expansion are turning down billions in federal funding that would flow into their states, support their hospitals, create healthcare jobs, and save lives—because accepting that funding would mean extending health coverage to poor people, disproportionately Black and Brown people, and the racist calculus says that's unacceptable.

This isn't about cost. It's not about state budgets. It's not about principled opposition to federal programs. If it were, these same states wouldn't eagerly accept other forms of federal funding. The opposition is specifically to healthcare coverage for poor people of color. The cruelty is the point. The suffering is the intended outcome.

During the 115th Congress (2017-2018), when ACA repeal was under active consideration, no states expanded Medicaid. The uncertainty about the ACA's future froze expansion efforts. States considering expansion held back because why expand if the federal funding and program structure might disappear? The threat of repeal had ripple effects beyond what was actually repealed—it prevented coverage expansion that would have happened otherwise.

This is how systemic racism operates in healthcare policy: not always through explicit racial language, but through deliberate policy choices that predictably harm people of color, made by politicians who understand exactly what they're doing and who they're harming. Medicaid expansion resistance is racist healthcare policy in action, no different in its fundamental cruelty than the segregated hospitals of the 1960s, just slightly more obscured by facially neutral language about "state flexibility" and "fiscal responsibility."

The states that refuse Medicaid expansion are the states that would benefit most from it. They have higher rates of poverty, worse health outcomes, and more residents who would gain coverage. They choose to leave their own residents uninsured rather than accept federal funding that would primarily help Black and Brown people. That choice is racism, structural and deliberate, killing people through policy.

The Repeated Attempts to Repeal

The Affordable Care Act became law in March 2010. Republicans began trying to repeal it immediately. Over the next fourteen years, they never stopped.

The most dramatic attempt came in 2017. Republicans controlled the House, Senate, and presidency. They'd campaigned for years on repealing "Obamacare." They finally had the power to do it. They tried.

The proposals varied in details but shared common elements: eliminate Medicaid expansion, eliminate marketplace premium tax credits, eliminate the individual mandate, slash Medicaid funding, allow states to waive essential health benefits requirements, permit insurance companies to charge older Americans far more than younger Americans, and generally dismantle the ACA's core protections.

The Congressional Budget Office estimated that the various repeal proposals would cause 23 to 32 million Americans to lose health insurance. Not might lose. Would lose. This wasn't speculation—it was mathematical certainty based on eliminating the programs and subsidies that made coverage possible for those millions of people.

Twenty-three to thirty-two million people. More than the entire population of Texas, and more than twice the population of Pennsylvania. An entire state's worth of people thrown off health insurance—not because they'd done anything wrong, not because they'd failed to pay premiums, but because Congress would eliminate the programs covering them.

The Republicans couldn't agree on which version of cruelty to enact. Some wanted immediate repeal. Others wanted delayed repeal. Some wanted to keep some ACA provisions. Others wanted complete elimination. They held votes. The proposals failed. They crafted new proposals. Those failed too.

The final vote came in July 2017. The Senate voted on "skinny repeal"—a scaled-back version that would still have eliminated the individual mandate and gutted the ACA's funding mechanisms. The vote was 49-51. It failed by one vote. John McCain—dying of brain cancer, understanding personally what healthcare crises look like—walked onto the Senate floor and gave a thumbs down that saved the ACA.

One vote. Twenty-three million people kept their health insurance because one senator voted no.

That's how close we came. That's how fragile the protections are. That's how many people's lives depend on the slimmest possible political margins.

The failure to repeal didn't end the attacks. If dramatic repeal wasn't possible, Republicans would pursue death by a thousand cuts. Administrative sabotage. Regulatory undermining. Funding cuts.

Each action designed to weaken the ACA incrementally, make coverage less accessible, drive people out of the marketplace, and create the appearance of ACA failure that could justify further attacks.

The Trump administration zeroed out the individual mandate penalty in 2017. The mandate required people to have insurance or pay a tax penalty—the mechanism that kept healthy people in the insurance pool and prevented adverse selection where only sick people buy coverage. Eliminating the penalty while keeping the mandate meant the requirement was unenforceable. Healthy people left the market. Premiums increased. The marketplace became less stable.

The Trump administration slashed funding for navigator programs by 90%—from $63 million to $10 million. Navigators are people who help consumers understand their insurance options, compare plans, and enroll in coverage. Eliminating navigator funding made enrollment harder, particularly for people with limited health insurance literacy, limited English proficiency, or limited internet access. Fewer people enrolled. The marketplace shrank.

The Trump administration canceled Healthcare.gov advertising. During open enrollment periods, the Obama administration ran extensive outreach campaigns to remind people that enrollment was happening and help them sign up. The Trump administration canceled those campaigns. Fewer people knew enrollment was happening, so fewer people enrolled.

The Trump administration shortened enrollment periods for the federal marketplace. Instead of three months to enroll, people got six weeks. This particularly hurt working people who needed time to compare plans, people with variable schedules, people who didn't realize enrollment was happening until it was almost over. Shorter enrollment meant fewer enrollments.

The cumulative effect: the effectiveness of ACA marketplace subsidies fell during the first Trump administration by more than 20% compared to the Obama years. Not because the subsidies changed—because administrative actions made it harder for people to access those subsidies. Enrollment dropped. Coverage declined. The ACA appeared to be failing, which was precisely the point. If you can't repeal a program, you sabotage it, then point to the sabotage as evidence the program doesn't work.

States using the federal marketplace platform were particularly vulnerable. Their residents experienced significant coverage declines between 2016 and 2019. States with their own state-based marketplaces proved more resilient—they maintained their own outreach, their own navigator programs, their own enrollment periods. State-based marketplaces have been twice as effective at expanding coverage per dollar of subsidy compared to federal platform states, largely because they're protected from federal administrative sabotage.

The Biden administration reversed the sabotage. Navigator funding increased to $100 million per year. Open enrollment periods lengthened. Healthcare.gov advertising resumed. Engagement with historically marginalized populations increased. The decline in marketplace effectiveness was fully reversed, even before accounting for the new subsidies from the American Rescue Plan.

But reversal requires constant vigilance and friendly administration. The sabotage can resume instantly whenever Republicans control the executive branch. The ACA survives not because it's secure but because people fight constantly to defend it from attack. Every election brings new threats. Every administration change brings potential new sabotage. The program that millions depend on exists in a state of permanent siege.

Work Requirements: Punishing the Poor for Being Poor

The first Trump administration approved thirteen state waivers for Medicaid work requirements before federal courts intervened. The Biden administration revoked these approvals, citing that work requirements reduced enrollment without promoting Medicaid's purpose of providing healthcare.

The second Trump administration didn't mess around with state waivers. They created a federal mandate.

The One Big Beautiful Bill Act, signed in 2025, requires all Medicaid expansion enrollees to work at least 80 hours per month or lose coverage beginning January 2027. Eligibility checks happen every 6 months instead of annually—with states allowed to check even more frequently.

The Congressional Budget Office estimates 10 million people will lose Medicaid by 2030, with 7.6 million becoming uninsured.

We know exactly what will happen because states have already tried this. Arkansas implemented work requirements in 2018. More than 95% of people who lost coverage were still eligible—they lost insurance because of administrative barriers, not because they weren't working. Employment among low-income adults? No change.

Georgia expanded Medicaid with work requirements in 2023. Compared to South Dakota, which expanded without work requirements at the same time, Georgia saw an 11.7 percentage point decrease in Medicaid coverage. Employment difference? Zero.

Work requirements don't increase employment. They create paperwork barriers that remove coverage from people who are already working or qualify for exemptions but can't prove it every 6 months.

The federal government just passed a law removing healthcare from 10 million people based on a policy that demonstrably doesn't work, using evidence from states that already proved it fails.

This isn't about encouraging work. It's about reducing Medicaid enrollment.

Work requirements sound reasonable on the surface: if you can work, you should work to earn your healthcare. The logic seems straightforward—taxpayers shouldn't pay for able-bodied adults who refuse to work.

That logic collapses instantly when you look at who Medicaid actually covers.

Children. They can't work. Medicaid covers approximately 40% of all children in America. Work requirements don't apply to children, but they affect children when their parents lose coverage for failing to meet paperwork requirements.

Elderly people. Many can't work due to age, disability, or health conditions. Medicaid covers long-term care for elderly Americans whose assets have been depleted by nursing home costs.

Disabled people. By definition, many cannot work or can only work limited hours. Medicaid is often their only access to healthcare and the services that allow them to survive.

People already working. The majority of non-disabled, non-elderly Medicaid recipients already work. They're earning poverty wages at jobs that don't provide health insurance. They're working part-time because they can't get full-time hours. They're cycling between jobs in the unstable low-wage labor market. They don't need incentives to work—they're already working as much as their circumstances allow.

Work requirements aren't about encouraging work. They're about creating bureaucratic barriers that kick people off coverage.

The requirements demand documentation: monthly reporting of work hours, proof of employment, verification of job search activities if unemployed, exemption applications for people who qualify for exemptions. The paperwork is complex. The deadlines are strict. The penalties for non-compliance are immediate loss of coverage.

People lose coverage not because they're not working but because they missed paperwork deadlines while working, couldn't navigate the complex reporting requirements, couldn't get their employer to provide documentation in time, didn't understand what was required, or couldn't access the reporting system. The bureaucratic barriers are the point—they're designed to reduce enrollment by making compliance difficult rather than by identifying people who genuinely refuse to work.

States that implemented work requirements saw coverage losses without corresponding employment gains. The requirements didn't make people work more. They just made people lose health insurance. Federal courts struck down several work requirement waivers, ruling that they violated Medicaid's statutory purpose of furnishing medical assistance to people who need it. Taking health insurance from poor people doesn't serve Medicaid's purpose—it subverts it.

Work requirements disproportionately affect Black and Brown people. They're concentrated in low-wage jobs with unstable hours, less likely to have jobs with flexibility to handle paperwork requirements, more likely to face discrimination in employment that makes finding and keeping work harder, and more likely to be living in poverty due to structural racism. Work requirements aren't race-neutral. They're racist policies by design, targeting people of color for coverage loss through facially neutral requirements that predictably harm them more.

The cruelty of work requirements is taking healthcare from people who need it most. The people on Medicaid are poor by definition—that's the eligibility criteria. They're struggling. They're working when they can, caring for family members, managing health conditions, navigating impossible economic circumstances. Work requirements add another impossible demand: document your deservingness monthly or lose the healthcare that keeps you alive.

Maria Rodriguez, whose story opened this chapter, was working. Sixteen hours per week. As much as her chronic conditions allowed. Not enough to meet the work requirement threshold. Not enough to prove she "deserved" healthcare. She lost coverage not because she was lazy or gaming the system but because the system was designed to exclude people exactly like her.

Work requirements embody American healthcare's moral bankruptcy: the belief that healthcare is something you must earn, that poor people don't deserve care unless they can prove their worthiness, that poverty is moral failure requiring punishment. This is evil. There's no other word for it. Taking healthcare from sick people and demanding they prove they deserve it by working enough hours is structural cruelty dressed up as reasonable policy.

What's Actually at Stake

The numbers are abstract until you understand what they represent. 40 million people covered by the ACA means forty million individuals, each with their own lives, families, health conditions, and futures that depend on having access to healthcare.

More than 21 million people have marketplace coverage as of 2024. These are people who don't have employer-sponsored insurance and don't qualify for Medicaid—often self-employed people, independent contractors, part-time workers, early retirees, people between jobs. Without marketplace subsidies, they couldn't afford insurance. Eliminate those subsidies and they become uninsured.

80 million people are covered by Medicaid, with expansion covering millions who'd previously been locked out of both Medicaid and affordable marketplace plans. These are the working poor, people with disabilities, children, and elderly people in nursing homes. Eliminate Medicaid expansion or slash Medicaid funding and tens of millions lose coverage.

Pre-existing condition protections affect 130+ million Americans who have conditions that would have been grounds for coverage denial pre-ACA. That's more than one-third of the American population. Most everyone has a pre-existing condition. Before the ACA, any of them could result in coverage denial or premiums so high they amounted to denial. Eliminate pre-existing condition protections and 130 million Americans face potential coverage loss or unaffordable premiums.

The provision allowing young adults to stay on parents' insurance until age 26 covers millions of people in their twenties who are establishing careers, often working jobs that don't provide insurance, and vulnerable to falling through coverage gaps. Eliminate this provision and young adults become the largest uninsured demographic again.

Essential health benefits requirements ensure insurance actually covers healthcare—hospitalization, emergency services, maternity care, mental health treatment, and prescription drugs. Before the ACA, plans could exclude entire categories of care. Allow states to waive essential health benefits and insurance coverage becomes illusory—you pay premiums for plans that don't cover the care you need.

The elimination of lifetime caps protects families facing catastrophic illness. Before the ACA, hitting your lifetime cap meant your insurance stopped paying for all future care. Children with complex medical needs, cancer patients, people with chronic conditions requiring ongoing expensive treatment—all vulnerable to hitting caps and becoming uninsured despite having paid premiums for years. Restore lifetime caps and families face financial catastrophe not just from high costs but from insurance literally ending when they need it most.

The prohibition on gender-based premium rating means women pay the same premiums as men. Before the ACA, being a woman cost you 50% more in premiums. Eliminate this protection and women again pay more for the crime of being female.

If the ACA is eliminated or substantially weakened, all of these protections disappear. Not gradually. Not with transition periods. Immediately. People lose coverage. Insurance companies can again deny coverage to sick people. Women pay more. Young adults become uninsured. Families hit lifetime caps and lose coverage. Medical bankruptcy increases beyond current catastrophic levels.

We know this because this is what existed before the ACA. This isn't speculation about what might happen. It's documented history of what did happen and what will happen again if protections are eliminated.

The human cost isn't abstract. It's people dying because they can't access care. It's families bankrupted by medical bills. It's children uninsured because their parents lost coverage. It's people with treatable conditions becoming disabled or dying because treatment is inaccessible. It's the cruelty of a system that decides healthcare is something only deserving people get to have.

The Medicaid Unwinding:
When Pandemic Protections Ended

During the COVID-19 pandemic, Congress required continuous enrollment in Medicaid—people couldn't be disenrolled for any reason except moving out of state. This kept people covered during a public health crisis when losing health insurance would have been catastrophic both for individuals and for pandemic response.

Medicaid enrollment increased by 23 million people between March 2020 and March 2023. Some of this growth came from people newly qualifying due to economic hardship during the pandemic. Much of it came from people who'd previously churned in and out of Medicaid remaining continuously enrolled. The continuous coverage requirement proved something important: when you eliminate bureaucratic barriers and keep people enrolled, coverage works. People stayed insured. They accessed care. The system functioned.

Then continuous enrollment ended in spring 2023.

States resumed eligibility redeterminations—the process of checking whether people still qualified for Medicaid and kicking off those who didn't. The "unwinding" began. Medicaid enrollment was projected to decline by 8.6% in fiscal year 2024.

The coverage losses weren't random. People lost coverage for two distinct reasons: genuine ineligibility (income increased above thresholds, moved out of state) and procedural reasons (missed paperwork deadlines, couldn't provide required documentation, didn't respond to notices in time). The procedural losses were particularly tragic—people who still qualified for Medicaid losing coverage because they couldn't navigate bureaucratic requirements.

Children lost coverage despite remaining eligible. Parents lost coverage, then forgot to re-enroll their children or didn't understand that children needed separate re-enrollment. States sent notices that went to old addresses. People working multiple jobs didn't have time to gather documentation within deadline windows. The bureaucratic barriers that work requirements deliberately create affected everyone during unwinding.

Fifteen million Americans lost Medicaid coverage. Many fell into the coverage gap in non-expansion states—too poor for subsidized marketplace plans, ineligible for Medicaid because their states refused expansion. Others became uninsured despite qualifying for marketplace subsidies because they didn't know subsidies existed or couldn't navigate enrollment.

Hospitals began seeing more uninsured patients. Emergency rooms filled with people who'd lost coverage and avoided care until conditions became critical. The preventable complications that insurance prevented began occurring again at higher rates.

The unwinding exposed the fragility of coverage. Even in a system that worked better during continuous enrollment, reintroducing bureaucratic barriers instantly threw millions off coverage. Many of those people still qualified for Medicaid—they just couldn't prove it fast enough or navigate the paperwork requirements. The system doesn't fail by denying coverage to ineligible people. It fails by making coverage so administratively complex that eligible people can't maintain it.

Despite the coverage losses, Medicaid take-up rates among eligible individuals remained surprisingly high during unwinding—86.5% in 2023 compared to 85.0% after the ACA (2017-2019) and 76.5% before the ACA (2008-2010). This persistence possibly reflects increased outreach efforts under the Biden administration that partially mitigated the bureaucratic barriers.

But 86.5% take-up means 13.5% of eligible people aren't enrolled. Millions of Americans qualify for Medicaid and aren't covered—not because they don't want coverage but because they can't navigate enrollment, don't know they qualify, or face barriers that prevent successful enrollment. Even a relatively high take-up rate means millions of eligible people remain uninsured.

The unwinding revealed what advocates have known all along: the administrative complexity that states build into Medicaid isn't accidental. It's designed to reduce enrollment. Continuous coverage worked. People stayed insured. When states reintroduced bureaucratic barriers, millions lost coverage. The barriers are the point. They exist to keep people off Medicaid, not to verify eligibility.

Current Threats and the Fight to Keep What We Have

The Affordable Care Act exists in a state of permanent siege. Every year brings new threats. Every administration change brings potential sabotage. Every legislative session brings bills to weaken, undermine, or repeal. The protections millions depend on are never secure.

The most recent major threat became reality: American Rescue Plan subsidies expired at the end of 2025 due to Congressional inaction. Without these enhanced subsidies, out-of-pocket premiums for the 22 million subsidized ACA enrollees increased by an average of 114%, or $1,016 per person. The Congressional Budget Office projected that 6.9 million fewer people would be enrolled in ACA Marketplace plans and 3.4 million more people would become uninsured. The largest premium increases hit older, middle-income enrollees—for example, a 60-year-old woman in Charlotte, North Carolina, making $64,000 saw her annual premium jump from $5,440 (8.5% of income) to $14,853 (23.2% of income).

These aren't just numbers—they're people forced to choose between paying rent and maintaining health insurance, people who will now avoid care, people who will develop preventable complications because coverage became unaffordable.

Additional legislative threats continue to loom, including proposals to eliminate the 90% federal match rate for Medicaid expansion. Currently, the federal government pays 90% of expansion costs. Proposed legislation would cut this to regular Medicaid matching rates (which vary by state but average around 60%). This would cut federal funding to expansion states by $44 billion annually, with a projected increase in the uninsured population of 10.8 million people.

Nine states have "trigger laws" that would automatically end their Medicaid expansions if the federal match rate drops, with three other states required to undergo automatic review. States couldn't afford to maintain expansion at regular match rates—the cost for all states to continue expanded Medicaid with a standard federal match would be $626 billion over a ten-year period. They'd end expansion. Everyone covered by expansion would lose insurance. The House Energy and Commerce Committee has been tasked with reducing federal spending by more than $800 billion over ten years, with most cuts expected to come from Medicaid.

Other proposed legislation would shift Medicaid from its current match-rate system to a per-capita allotment—giving states a fixed amount per enrollee rather than matching state spending. Per-capita caps would cut federal Medicaid funding, forcing states to either cut benefits, restrict eligibility, reduce provider payments (driving providers out of Medicaid), or make up the difference with state funds they don't have. The result: coverage losses, reduced benefits, fewer providers accepting Medicaid, deteriorating access to care.

Administrative threats include proposed "marketplace integrity and affordability" rules that would reverse Biden-era policies that streamlined enrollment and gave people more time to sign up. The proposed rules would shorten open enrollment from 75 days to 45 days, put consumers auto-renewed for $0 plans into plans with a $5 monthly premium until they confirm eligibility, make it harder for low-income individuals to enroll midyear, and force state-based marketplaces to use the new 45-day period, eliminating the autonomy that made state-based marketplaces twice as effective at expanding coverage per dollar of subsidy. These changes would recreate the Trump-era sabotage that the Biden administration reversed—Biden policies had made subsidies more than 30% more effective than during the first Trump term.

Navigator funding was slashed by 90% in February 2025—from $100 million back down to $10 million. This eliminated most of the people who help consumers enroll in coverage, particularly affecting people with limited health insurance literacy, limited English proficiency, rural residents, and historically marginalized populations. Fewer navigators mean fewer enrollments mean more uninsured people.

Legislative proposals continue circulating that would repeal the Biden administration's fix to the "family glitch"—a provision that made some dependents ineligible for marketplace subsidies even though family coverage through an employer was unaffordable. The Biden fix extended subsidies to these dependents. Repealing it would exclude them from subsidies again, making coverage unaffordable.

Additional administrative barriers were added through legislation in November 2025 requiring income verification before enrollment, targeting what the administration called "phantom patients"—an estimated 6.4 million enrollees who either were allegedly ineligible or did not know they had coverage. This new verification requirement adds another bureaucratic hurdle that will inevitably exclude eligible people who can't quickly provide required documentation.

Each threat affects millions of people. Each represents coverage losses, increased costs, reduced access to care, more medical bankruptcies, more preventable deaths. The threats aren't theoretical—they're legislative proposals, regulatory actions, and administrative decisions actively being pursued and, in some cases, already implemented.

The pattern is consistent: every threat benefits insurance companies, reduces government healthcare spending, and harms patients. The threats don't come from nowhere—they're pushed by industry lobbying that prioritizes profit over people, by politicians funded by healthcare industry campaign contributions, by ideological opposition to any government role in healthcare regardless of human cost.

The ACA survives through constant defensive fighting. Healthcare advocates spend all their energy preventing coverage losses rather than advancing toward universal coverage. Every legislative session brings the same battles: fighting to extend or restore subsidies, fighting to preserve Medicaid expansion, fighting to stop benefit cuts, fighting to maintain navigator funding, fighting to prevent administrative sabotage.

This exhaustion is strategic. Keep advocates defending inadequate programs so they can't organize for adequate ones. Keep the fight focused on "preserve ACA vs. eliminate ACA" so it never becomes "ACA vs. universal healthcare." Keep people afraid of losing what little they have so they can't demand better.

The system works perfectly. Not for patients—for the industries profiting from patient suffering. As long as the fight is "keep inadequate protections vs. eliminate them," industry wins regardless of outcome. If protections are eliminated, industry profits from less regulation. If protections survive, they're too weak to threaten industry profits. Either way, the real solution—universal healthcare that eliminates insurance company profit extraction—never gets serious consideration.

Fighting for Scraps of Dignity

The Affordable Care Act represents bare minimum human decency: insurance companies can't deny coverage to sick people, can't kick people off when they get expensive, can't charge women more for being women, must cover essential health benefits, and can't impose lifetime caps. These aren't radical demands. They're the baseline requirements for insurance to be insurance rather than a scam that takes premiums while you're healthy and denies coverage when you're sick.

This is what Americans are reduced to fighting for. Not universal healthcare. Not single-payer. Not the comprehensive coverage that every other developed nation guarantees as a human right. Just basic protections against insurance company cruelty. Just the minimum decency of "don't deny coverage to people with pre-existing conditions."

Still, even these minimal protections are under constant attack.

Americans fight to preserve inadequacy rather than fighting for actual solutions. Every ounce of energy spent defending the ACA is energy not available for advancing universal healthcare. Every political battle over keeping Medicaid expansion is a battle not fought over Medicare for All. The defensive crutch becomes permanent.

This is what it means to fight for scraps of dignity: celebrating when you successfully prevent coverage losses rather than demanding coverage that works. Being grateful for high-deductible insurance that still bankrupts you because at least you have something. Accepting medical debt, job lock, surprise bills, and provider burnout as inevitable rather than demanding a system that doesn't generate these cruelties by design.

The exhaustion is profound. Healthcare advocates have been fighting Republican repeal attempts since 2010—fifteen years of constant defensive battles. The victories are preventing things from getting worse, never making things actually good. Win after win that keeps the system inadequate rather than advancing toward adequacy.

As you know, I work in this system. I have coverage through the ACA marketplace. I've benefited from pre-existing condition protections that would have denied or priced me out of coverage before 2014. I'm grateful these protections exist. I'm also furious that Americans have to fight constantly to preserve them, that having to change insurance carriers every few years due to cost or carriers dropping coverage is considered normal, that paying outrageous premiums for high-deductible plans is the best we can do, and that even with ACA protections people still go bankrupt from medical debt and die from lack of care.

The ACA helped millions of people. It's also a compromise that preserved industry profits while adding minimal regulations. It's simultaneously too important to lose and too inadequate to accept as the final answer. Both things are true. The fight to keep inadequate protections is necessary. It's also tragic that this is what American healthcare politics have become: fighting for scraps while every other developed nation guarantees healthcare as a human right.

The System Working As Designed

The Affordable Care Act under constant siege isn't an accident. It's not unfortunate political polarization or honest policy disagreement. It's a deliberate strategy to keep American healthcare dysfunctional enough to maximize profit while preventing the reforms that would actually solve problems.

Keep the ACA weak enough that problems persist—medical bankruptcy continues, people avoid care due to cost, fragmentation kills, and providers burn out. Blame the ACA for problems that exist because it wasn't allowed to go far enough. Use the problems it didn't solve as justification for repealing the minimal protections it did create.

Keep the ACA under constant threat so advocates spend all their energy defending rather than advancing. Exhaust the people who would organize for universal healthcare by forcing them to fight repeatedly to preserve inadequate coverage. Make every political cycle a battle over whether to keep or eliminate the ACA so the conversation never advances to "what system would actually work."

This serves industry interests perfectly. Insurance companies get to keep profiting with minimal regulation. Pharmaceutical companies face no price controls. Hospitals maintain their pricing power. The ACA's regulations are annoying to industry but not threatening—they're workarounds, not fundamental challenges to the profit-extraction model.

The political theater of repeal attempts distracts from real solutions. As long as the debate is "keep ACA or repeal it," the debate is never "ACA or universal healthcare." Industry benefits from both options: elimination would remove regulations, preservation maintains profit-driven structure. What industry can't tolerate is the conversation shifting to single-payer systems that would eliminate insurance company profits entirely.

So the ACA remains under attack. Not because it failed—it helped millions of people. It's under attack because helping millions of people while preserving industry profits is exactly the outcome industry wants to maintain. They want it weak enough to leave problems the industry can profit from, and strong enough that people fear losing it, fighting to preserve it rather than demanding better.

The coverage losses, the bureaucratic barriers, the administrative sabotage, the legislative threats—all of it serves to keep American healthcare broken in ways that generate profit. The system doesn't fail. It works exactly as designed: extracting maximum revenue while providing minimum care, keeping patients afraid and advocates exhausted, ensuring that the conversation never advances from "preserve inadequate protections" to "demand adequate ones."

The Affordable Care Act is sick by design—designed to be better than what came before but worse than what's needed; designed to help some people while leaving fundamental problems intact; designed to be under permanent threat so improvements seem impossible. This is American healthcare policy: fighting for scraps of dignity while the rest of the developed world guarantees healthcare as a human right and wonders why Americans accept such cruelty as normal.

> *At this point, you might look to someone like me—a healthcare provider—and ask: how can you work within a system like this? To be perfectly honest, many of us can't. The cruelty of the American healthcare system affects all of us—including those working within it.*

CHAPTER

10 From the Wrong Side

The Physician Who Quit

The following scenario is a composite constructed from common patterns observed among healthcare workers experiencing moral injury. The details are hypothetical, but the dynamics are real and pervasive in American healthcare.

Dr. Sophia Brown had wanted to be a doctor since she was eight years old. She'd made it through medical school, survived residency, built a successful primary care practice. She was good at her job—thorough, compassionate, and evidence-based. Her patients loved her. Her colleagues respected her. By every conventional measure, she was a successful physician.

At forty-two, she quit medicine entirely.

Not because she was tired. Not because the hours were too long or the work too demanding. She quit because she couldn't participate in the harm anymore.

The breaking point came on a Tuesday afternoon. A patient with advanced diabetes needed a newer medication that would significantly improve her blood sugar control and reduce her risk of kidney failure. Sophia wrote the prescription. The insurance company denied it. Not because the medication wasn't medically necessary—it clearly was. Not because Sophia hadn't provided sufficient documentation—she'd submitted detailed clinical notes, lab results, and peer-reviewed evidence supporting her choice. The insurance company denied it because the patient hadn't "failed" on two cheaper medications first.

Sophia knew those cheaper medications wouldn't work as well. She knew the patient's kidney function was already declining. She knew that delaying effective treatment would likely result in permanent kidney damage. She also knew the insurance company didn't care.

She spent two hours on the phone that afternoon—two hours she should have spent seeing patients—arguing with insurance company representatives who weren't clinicians, who had never examined this patient, who were reading from scripts designed to maximize denials. She escalated to a "peer-to-peer" review with an insurance company physician who spent three minutes on the call before upholding the denial.

The patient would have to fail on inferior medications—medications Sophia knew wouldn't adequately control her diabetes—before insurance would cover the medication she actually needed. By the time the patient "failed" sufficiently to satisfy the insurance company's requirements, her kidneys would be irreversibly damaged.

Sophia prescribed the inferior medication. She watched her patient's blood sugar remain poorly controlled. She watched the kidney function tests worsen. She documented everything carefully, building the case for the inevitable appeal when the cheaper medication failed to work.

She did her job. She followed the rules. She participated in harming her patient because the system required it.

That night, Sophia sat in her car in the clinic parking lot and cried. Not from exhaustion—from moral devastation. She'd spent two hours fighting for her patient and lost. She'd prescribed medication she knew was inadequate. She'd watched a preventable complication begin unfolding in slow motion, powerless to stop it because an insurance company employee with no medical training had overruled her clinical judgment.

This wasn't the first time. It happened weekly, sometimes daily. Insurance denials for necessary care. Prior authorizations that took hours to complete. Formulary restrictions that forced her to prescribe inferior medications. Patients who couldn't afford co-pays for the treatments they needed. Fifteen-minute appointment slots for patients with complex problems requiring an hour. Corporate productivity metrics that measured how many patients she saw, not whether they got better.

Sophia had spent fifteen years becoming an excellent physician. The system had spent fifteen years forcing her to participate in substandard, harmful care. She was complicit in a machine designed to maximize profit by minimizing the care her patients received. Every day, she watched people suffer because insurance companies and corporate healthcare administrators prioritized money over health. Every day, she was forced to be the face of that cruelty.

The exhaustion she could have handled. The long hours, the difficult diagnoses, the patients who didn't get better despite her best efforts—

those were part of medicine, and she'd accepted them. What she couldn't accept was being forced to harm patients by a system designed to deny them the care they needed.

She quit three months later. No dramatic exit, no public statement. She just stopped seeing patients, walked away from a career she'd spent two decades building. Her colleagues were shocked. Her patients were devastated. The system didn't notice. There were plenty of other physicians to exploit.

Sophia now works in medical education, teaching but not practicing. She still loves medicine. She can't bear to practice it. The moral injury was too deep. Being forced to participate in systematic harm had broken something in her that couldn't be repaired while staying in clinical practice.

She's not alone. Thousands of healthcare workers are leaving clinical practice every year—not because they don't care, but because they care too much to keep participating in a system designed to harm the people they're trying to help.

Burnout vs. Moral Injury: Understanding the Difference

Healthcare worker suffering is often described as "burnout," but that word obscures what's actually happening. Burnout implies that providers are tired, overworked, depleted—that they need better self-care, more resilience training, maybe some yoga and meditation. This framing locates the problem in individual providers rather than in the system that's destroying them.

Moral injury is different. More accurate. More honest about what the system does to healthcare workers.

Burnout is exhaustion from working too hard with insufficient resources. Long shifts, inadequate staffing, overwhelming patient loads, administrative burdens that consume time better spent on patient care. These are real problems. They contribute to provider suffering. However, they're not the whole story, and focusing only on burnout obscures the deeper harm.

Moral injury is psychological and spiritual damage that occurs when you're forced to participate in actions that violate your core values and professional commitments. It's what happens when the system requires you to be complicit in harm you can recognize but can't prevent.

For healthcare workers, moral injury means:

- Being forced to deny care you know patients need because insurance companies won't cover it.
- Being forced to discharge hospital patients before they're stable because insurance won't authorize additional days.
- Being forced to prescribe inferior medications because formularies exclude more effective drugs.
- Being forced to rush through fifteen-minute appointments with complex patients who need an hour of your time.
- Being forced to prioritize documentation and billing over actual patient care.
- Being forced to watch patients suffer from preventable complications because the system prioritizes profit over health.

Most devastatingly, being forced to be the face of these failures—to be the person who has to tell patients their insurance denied coverage, who has to explain why they can't have the medication they need, who has to discharge them before they're ready, who becomes in patients' eyes the representative of a cruel system the provider has no power to change.

The distinguishing feature of moral injury isn't exhaustion. It's being forced to violate your professional ethics and personal values repeatedly, systematically, as a requirement of continued employment. Healthcare workers don't just get tired. They get morally wounded by being made complicit in harm they're trained to prevent.

The system deliberately creates this injury. Healthcare workers enter the field to help people. The system then structures their work to ensure they regularly participate in harming people—through denials, through inadequate time, through cost-based rationing, through all the mechanisms that prioritize profit over care. This isn't accidental. Exhausted, demoralized, morally injured healthcare workers are easier to control. They're less likely to organize for systemic change. They're more likely to accept the system as it is because they lack the energy and hope needed to fight it.

Moral injury serves the system's interests. Burned out providers might quit, but they'll be replaced. Morally injured providers stay in place, wounded and complicit, continuing to participate in the harm because they have student loan debt, families to support, and nowhere else to go. The system needs their complicity. So it creates conditions that guarantee moral injury while calling it burnout and offering resilience training instead of systemic change.

The Scale of the Crisis

The statistics on healthcare worker suffering are catastrophic and getting worse.

Current physician burnout rates hover around 48-53%, with more than half of practicing physicians and trainees experiencing burnout. What these numbers obscure is the severity of the crisis because they fluctuate based on external stressors while the underlying trend is clear: healthcare workers are being systematically destroyed by the conditions under which they're forced to practice.

In 2017, physician burnout was 43.9%. It dropped to 38.2% in 2020, creating false hope that things were improving. Then the COVID-19 pandemic hit and burnout surged to 62.8% in 2021. By 2022 it had declined to 53.0%, and by 2023 to 48.2%—still higher than 2017, still affecting nearly half of all physicians.

These fluctuations track with acute stressors like pandemic conditions, but they mask the chronic underlying crisis. The system wasn't working well in 2017 when burnout was "only" 44%. It wasn't fixed in 2020 when rates temporarily improved. The fundamental conditions creating moral injury—insurance denials, time pressure, corporate control, profit prioritization—remained constant throughout these fluctuations.

The broader healthcare workforce shows even worse numbers. Among all healthcare workers, burnout increased from 67.9% in 2018 to 79.1% in 2022. Nearly four out of five healthcare workers are burned out. This isn't a few struggling individuals who need better coping strategies. This is wholesale workforce destruction.

Nurses show burnout rates notably higher than several physician specialties. Mental health professionals—psychiatrists, psychologists, social workers—show particularly high burnout rates, which is darkly ironic given that these are the professionals theoretically equipped to handle psychological stress. Even they can't withstand the moral injury of practicing in a system designed to harm patients.

Burnout varies by specialty and setting. Emergency medicine and intensive care show elevated rates—perhaps unsurprisingly given the high-acuity, high-stress nature of the work. The problem becomes apparent when general practitioners, who theoretically have more control over their schedules and lower-acuity patients, also show substantial burnout. The issue isn't just the inherent difficulty of medical work. It's the system within which that work occurs.

The mental health toll extends beyond burnout. Depression affects approximately 33% of physicians—one in three. Anxiety affects 24%. PTSD affects 10%. These rates are substantially elevated compared to the general population. Healthcare workers aren't inherently more prone to mental illness. The conditions under which they work create mental illness.

Suicidal ideation affects 6-14% of physicians and trainees, with current rates around 10%. One in ten physicians has recently considered suicide. Among those, 1-2.5% have attempted suicide. These aren't statistics about a struggling fringe. These are numbers that should trigger immediate, comprehensive systemic intervention.

Certain specialties face particularly elevated suicide risk: anesthesiologists, general practitioners, psychiatrists, and general surgeons. The specialties vary, but the pattern is consistent—healthcare workers across all domains are suffering mental health crises at rates that would be considered catastrophic in any other profession.

The consequences extend beyond individual suffering to workforce retention. Compared to physicians without burnout, those experiencing burnout have more than threefold increased odds of turnover intention and more than threefold increased career choice regret. Job satisfaction decreases nearly fourfold. Healthcare workers who are burned out and morally injured don't just suffer—they leave. They quit clinical practice, retire early, or stay physically present while mentally checking out.

The proportion of physicians reporting burnout symptoms decreased from 45.5% in 2011 to 38.0% in 2020, and this decrease corresponded with a decrease in work hours. This suggests that workload reduction helps—but it also reveals the trap. The only way to reduce burnout in the current system is to work less, see fewer patients, and provide less care. The system's solution to provider suffering is to reduce the amount of healthcare provided. This is not a solution. It's an admission that the system cannot sustain adequate healthcare delivery without destroying the people who provide it.

The crisis is particularly severe among younger physicians and women. Female physicians show higher burnout rates than male physicians across most studies. Burnout peaks during training and mid-career—the periods when physicians are most heavily exploited by the system, working the longest hours with the least autonomy and the greatest debt burden.

These aren't just statistics about individual suffering. They're evidence of systematic workforce destruction. American healthcare is consuming and discarding the people who make it function. We're burning through healthcare workers at rates that cannot be sustained, then wondering why there are workforce shortages and why the people who remain are increasingly demoralized and detached.

The system is working exactly as designed. Exhausted, morally injured, psychologically damaged healthcare workers serve the system's interests by being too broken to organize for change, too trapped by debt and obligations to leave, and too demoralized to believe anything can be different.

What Creates Moral Injury: The Daily Cruelty

Moral injury doesn't result from single traumatic events. It accumulates through daily exposure to systemic cruelty that healthcare workers are forced to participate in and cannot prevent.

The insurance denial machine operates continuously. Prior authorizations are required for basic, evidence-based medical care. A primary care physician wants to order an MRI for a patient with neurological symptoms suggesting a serious condition. Before the MRI can be scheduled, the physician or their staff must contact the insurance company, provide detailed clinical information, and justify why the test is medically necessary. This process takes anywhere from fifteen minutes to several hours depending on the insurance company's responsiveness and requirements.

The insurance company reviews the request—not immediately, but within their processing timeframe, which can be days or weeks. During this time, the patient waits. The concerning symptoms continue. The physician worries. If the patient's condition worsens during the delay, that harm falls on the patient while the insurance company faces no consequences for delaying necessary diagnostic testing.

Many prior authorization requests are approved—but only after wasting hours of staff time that could have been spent on patient care. The prior authorization requirement serves no medical purpose. It exists purely to create friction, to make ordering tests and treatments more difficult, and to discourage physicians from ordering care that might cost the insurance company money.

Some prior authorizations are denied. The insurance company decides—based on policies written by administrators, not on clinical evaluation of the actual patient—that the test or treatment isn't "medically necessary." The physician can appeal, spending more hours providing additional documentation and arguing with insurance company representatives who follow scripts designed to uphold denials. Most appeals fail.

In Medicare Advantage plans, private insurers made nearly 50 million prior authorization determinations in 2023, with 6.4% fully or partially denied. That's 3.2 million denials in a single year in Medicare Advantage alone. In ACA marketplace plans, 20% of claims were denied in 2023. One in five. These aren't edge cases or questionable treatments. These are denials of care that physicians determined was medically necessary.

Healthcare workers live with this constantly. Every day brings insurance denials for necessary care. Diabetic patients can't get the medications that would best control their disease because insurance requires "step therapy"—forcing patients to fail on cheaper, less effective medications before covering better ones. I've had multiple diabetic patients tell me their insurance wouldn't cover Ozempic despite it being prescribed for diabetes management. One patient was denied without explanation, likely because medication shortages driven by off-label use for weight loss made insurance companies even more restrictive about covering it for its approved indication.

The cruelty is deliberate. Step therapy doesn't exist for clinical reasons—it exists to save insurance companies money by forcing patients onto cheaper medications even when more expensive medications are more effective. The system requires physicians to prescribe medications they know are inferior, watch their patients' conditions remain poorly controlled, document the "failure" of the inadequate medication, and then fight through another prior authorization process to get the medication that should have been prescribed initially.

Meanwhile, the patient suffers. Their diabetes isn't adequately controlled. They're at higher risk for complications—kidney disease, blindness, amputations, heart attacks, and strokes. All preventable with proper medication management. All occurring anyway because insurance companies profit from denying effective care.

Formulary restrictions compound the problem. Insurance companies maintain lists of "approved" medications—formularies that exclude many effective treatments in favor of cheaper alternatives. When a physician prescribes a medication not in the formulary, it's not covered. The patient either pays out of pocket—often hundreds or thousands of dollars they don't have—or they take the inferior formulary medication.

Patients constantly ask about medication costs. This is routine now, normalized to the point where it barely registers as the obscenity it is. Patients need to know if they can afford the medication their physician is prescribing. Providers have learned to check formularies before prescribing, to consult with pharmacists about cheaper alternatives, to prescribe based on what insurance will cover rather than on what will work best.

This is treating insurance companies' financial interests instead of treating patients. Providers are forced to make clinical decisions based on cost rather than effectiveness. They know they're providing suboptimal care. They have no choice. The alternative is prescribing medications patients can't afford and won't take, which is even worse than prescribing medications that work less well but are covered by insurance.

The time restrictions create a different form of cruelty. Fifteen-minute appointment slots for patients with complex, chronic conditions requiring comprehensive evaluation and management. Providers are expected to review the patient's history, perform an examination, order appropriate tests, make diagnoses, develop treatment plans, provide patient education, document everything thoroughly for billing and legal purposes, and somehow also build a therapeutic relationship—all in fifteen minutes or less.

It's impossible. Everyone knows it's impossible. Providers do it anyway because productivity metrics demand it. Corporate employers and insurance reimbursement models pay based on volume—how many patients seen, not how well they're cared for. Providers who spend thirty minutes with complex patients see half as many patients, generate half as much revenue, and get penalized for "low productivity."

I worked in an occupational health and urgent care clinic where we saw walk-in patients all day. Back-to-back appointments with fifteen-minute slots. You were incentivized to see patients quickly—not explicitly penalized for taking longer, but the patient volume was so high that if you wanted to leave work on time, you had to keep moving. I routinely worked past 5 p.m., seeing patients after the clinic officially closed because there was no other way to get through the volume.

The work was relentlessly stressful. No breaks. No time to think. Just patient after patient after patient, each with problems requiring more time and attention than the schedule allowed. Complex patients got superficial care, not because I didn't care, but because the system allotted fifteen minutes and there were ten more patients waiting.

This creates moral injury not because the work is hard—providers expect hard work—but because you know you're providing inadequate care. You know the patient needs more time. You know you're missing things in the rush. You know you're not building the kind of therapeutic relationship that facilitates good outcomes. You know all of this, and you keep doing it anyway because the alternative is losing your job.

The electronic health record intensifies the time pressure. EHR systems are designed for billing, not clinical care. Every click must be documented. Every diagnosis must be coded. Every intervention must be captured for billing purposes. Providers spend more time clicking boxes in the EHR than talking to patients. They make eye contact with computer screens instead of with the people they're treating.

The documentation burden is crushing. After seeing patients all day, providers spend hours in the evening completing notes, responding to electronic messages, reviewing test results, and managing prescription refills. The clinical day never ends. The EHR follows providers home, demanding attention during time that should be spent with family, resting, living a life outside of medicine.

The use of scribes—people who handle EHR documentation while providers focus on patients—has been shown to substantially improve productivity and provider satisfaction. The addition of clerical support consistently improves provider well-being. This tells us something important: the problem isn't medicine, it's the administrative burden imposed by systems designed to maximize billing rather than optimize care.

Corporate medicine strips autonomy. Increasingly, providers work as employees of large healthcare corporations rather than in independent practices. Corporate employers impose policies prioritizing profit: productivity quotas, patient satisfaction scores (tied to reimbursement, not to quality of care), formulary restrictions, limitations on testing, and requirements to see patients in inadequate time slots.

Providers have no meaningful input into these policies. Administrators with no clinical training make decisions about how medicine should be practiced. Providers who object, who advocate for their patients, who push back against policies that compromise care, get threatened with termination.

The loss of professional autonomy is profound. Healthcare providers—physicians, nurse practitioners, physician assistants—train for years to develop clinical judgment. Then they're employed by corporations that don't trust that judgment, that override clinical decisions for financial reasons, that treat providers as interchangeable widgets in a profit-generating machine.

Every day, healthcare workers are forced to participate in this cruelty. Every day, they watch patients suffer from denials, from inadequate time, from cost-based rationing, from administrative policies that prioritize money over health. Every day, they're complicit in a system designed to harm the people they're trying to help.

This is moral injury. Not exhaustion from working hard—everyone expected that. It's being forced to violate your core professional values repeatedly, systematically, as a condition of continued employment. It's watching people suffer when you know how to help them but the system won't let you. It's participating in harm because refusing to participate means losing your job, defaulting on your student loans, losing your ability to support your family.

The cruelty is structural, deliberate, and profitable. It's destroying the healthcare workforce one morally injured provider at a time.

How the System Weaponizes Providers Against Patients

One of the most insidious mechanisms of moral injury is how the system forces healthcare workers to be the face of institutional cruelty they don't control and can't prevent.

When insurance denies coverage, it's the provider who has to deliver the bad news. The patient doesn't see the insurance company executive who designed the denial policy or the claims adjuster who processed the denial. They see their provider—the person they trusted to help them—telling them they can't have the treatment they need.

"Your insurance won't cover this." Five words that providers say constantly, knowing that patients often hear them as "I won't help you" rather than "A corporation you pay premiums to is refusing to cover necessary care."

The patient's anger, fear, and desperation get directed at the provider. The insurance company remains invisible. The provider becomes the villain in the patient's experience even though the provider is fighting for the patient and losing to a system designed to deny care.

I have these conversations constantly. Patients needing care that insurance wouldn't cover. Explaining why I couldn't order the test they needed, couldn't prescribe the medication that would work best. Having to be the person who said no when I desperately wanted to say yes.

Most patients understood. I often had frank conversations with patients about how broken the American healthcare system is, and most agreed. They knew the system was designed to extract money while providing minimal care. They knew insurance companies and corporate healthcare profited while patients suffered. They knew providers were trapped in the same system.

However, this understanding doesn't eliminate the harm. Even when patients know intellectually that their provider isn't the problem, emotionally they're still sitting in an exam room with a provider who's telling them they can't have what they need. The provider becomes associated with denial, with inadequacy, with failure—even when the provider is doing everything possible within an impossible system.

This erosion of trust between patients and providers serves the system's interests. If patients and providers united against the insurance companies and corporations exploiting them both, they'd be a powerful force for change. So the system keeps them divided. Patients see providers as the face of denial. Providers see patients as yet another person they're failing, yet another interaction where they're forced to participate in harm.

The system ensures that when things go wrong, providers bear the consequences. Patients sue providers for malpractice when poor outcomes result from insurance denials or inadequate time or systemic failures beyond the provider's control. The insurance companies and corporations that created those conditions face no legal liability. The provider who tried to provide good care within impossible constraints becomes legally responsible for the predictable failures that result.

Hospital discharge is a particularly cruel example. Insurance authorizes a certain number of hospital days. When those days expire, the patient must be discharged regardless of whether they're medically ready. Physicians know the patient isn't stable, that they need more time, and that early discharge will likely result in readmission or complications. The insurance company doesn't care. Continued hospitalization won't be paid. The patient must leave.

The physician has to discharge a patient they know isn't ready. They have to explain to the patient—who feels terrible, who's frightened, who can see they're not well enough to go home—that they're being sent home anyway. The patient doesn't blame the insurance company. They blame the physician and hospital for "kicking them out." The physician experiences the moral injury of participating in harm while also receiving the patient's anger about that harm.

When patients end up back in the emergency room or hospital within days of discharge—which happens predictably when patients are discharged too early—it looks like a failure of the discharging physician rather than a failure of insurance policies that prioritize cost over care. The physician's reputation suffers. The hospital's readmission rates increase, triggering Medicare penalties. The insurance company that forced the early discharge faces no consequences.

Providers become trapped between corporate policies they can't control and patients who need the care those policies deny. I had a young man in his thirties tell me he had unexplained rectal bleeding. I knew he needed a colonoscopy—colon cancer is occurring at younger and younger ages, and unexplained rectal bleeding requires evaluation. I also knew that if I ordered the colonoscopy directly, insurance likely wouldn't cover it because he didn't meet their criteria. The best I could do was refer him to gastroenterology and let them order the colonoscopy.

This delay—sending him to a specialist who would then order the test I already knew he needed—serves no medical purpose. It increases costs (specialist visit plus procedure instead of just procedure), delays diagnosis, and puts the patient at risk while we wait for insurance approval. On the other hand, ordering the colonoscopy directly would likely result in denial and the patient receiving a bill for thousands of dollars.

So I participated in the delay. I referred to the specialist. I documented my concerns. I did what the system allowed me to do. As a result, I lived with the knowledge that if this young man had colon cancer, the delay I was forced to create could affect his outcome. The system made me complicit in potentially harming him while making it look like I was following proper procedures.

This is how the system weaponizes providers. It forces them to be the face of harmful policies. It ensures that when patients are hurt by cost-based rationing, insurance denials, and corporate profit maximization, they direct their anger and distrust at individual providers rather than at the system creating the harm. It makes providers feel personally responsible for systemic failures they're powerless to prevent.

The psychological impact is devastating. Providers enter healthcare to help people. The system forces them to harm people while making them appear to be the agents of that harm. They become the bad guys in their patients' stories even though they're fighting for their patients and losing to corporations that don't care.

This division serves the system perfectly. As long as patients see providers as the problem, and providers see themselves as failures, neither group organizes effectively for systemic change. The insurance companies and corporate healthcare systems continue profiting while patients and providers blame each other for suffering both are experiencing at the hands of a system designed to maximize extraction while minimizing care.

The Racial Dynamics of Provider Complicity

Moral injury is compounded for healthcare workers forced to practice within structurally racist systems. White providers participate daily in segregated care systems that deliver inferior treatment to Black and Brown patients. Providers of color witness racism against their patients while also experiencing racism themselves within hierarchical healthcare institutions. All healthcare workers become complicit in perpetuating racial health inequities they recognize but cannot individually fix.

The segregation in American healthcare operates through insurance status, which correlates strongly with race. Black and Latino patients are more likely to have Medicaid or be uninsured compared to White patients. Healthcare systems concentrate resources in well-insured (predominantly White) populations while providing separate, inferior care to Medicaid patients and the uninsured (disproportionately patients of color).

Clinics serving predominantly Medicaid populations have fewer resources, longer wait times, higher staff turnover, and lower-paid providers. Medicaid patients get referred to resident clinics staffed by trainees rather than experienced physicians. They receive less access to specialists, longer delays for diagnostic testing, and are offered less aggressive treatment options.

Providers working in these segregated systems witness daily how Black and Brown patients receive worse care. They see the under-resourced clinics, the overbooked schedules, the limited treatment options. They know that if these same patients had private insurance, they'd have better access to specialists, newer medications, more comprehensive care. But the system is designed this way, with financial incentives that direct resources toward privately insured patients and away from Medicaid populations.

Individual providers can't fix this. A physician working in a Medicaid clinic can provide the best care possible within that setting, but they can't change the fact that the setting itself has fewer resources, less support staff, more restrictive formularies, and limited specialist access compared to private practices serving well-insured patients. They participate in unequal care by working within these structurally unequal systems.

I once had a young Black woman come to urgent care. Based on her symptoms, I suspected a pulmonary embolism—a blood clot in the lungs that can be fatal if not treated immediately. A White physician in the clinic had seen her first and blown her off, telling me it couldn't be a PE because her oxygen saturation was normal. He pushed her care onto me— a Black nurse practitioner, thank goodness.

I knew he was wrong. Normal oxygen saturations don't rule out PE. Her symptoms—shortness of breath, chest pain, young age, race—were concerning. I called an ambulance. I insisted that everyone—the EMTs, her friend, the patient herself—knew what I suspected before she went to the hospital. I made sure they understood this was potentially life-threatening and needed immediate evaluation.

She called me a few days later. She'd had a pulmonary embolism. The hospital had confirmed it. She thanked me for saving her life.

This is the racial dynamic of American healthcare in miniature: a White physician dismissing a young Black woman's symptoms as not serious. A Black woman whose concerning symptoms almost got inadequate treatment because the first provider didn't take her seriously. The reality that if I hadn't been there, if I hadn't insisted, if I hadn't made sure everyone understood the urgency, she might have died from a treatable condition because a White physician didn't believe her symptoms warranted aggressive evaluation.

How many Black patients present with serious symptoms that get dismissed? How many die or suffer preventable complications because providers—even well-meaning ones—don't take Black patients' symptoms as seriously as they would White patients' symptoms? The research shows this happens systematically. Black patients' pain is undertreated. Their symptoms are dismissed as exaggerated. They receive less aggressive care for the same conditions.

Providers of color experience additional layers of moral injury. They witness racism against their patients while also experiencing racism within healthcare institutions. They see how White patients get preferential treatment. They watch Black and Brown patients get inferior care. They know that their own race affects how they're treated by colleagues, how much authority they're granted, whether their clinical judgment is respected.

They carry the burden of being expected to care for patients of color—as if matching race resolves the structural inequities in care delivery—while simultaneously facing discrimination within predominantly White healthcare institutions that undervalue and underpay providers of color. They experience the exhaustion of fighting institutional racism while trying to provide good patient care within systems designed to perpetuate racial health inequities.

The moral injury is knowing that the system you work within is racist, seeing how that racism harms patients daily, and being unable to fix it because the racism is structural rather than individual. You can provide excellent care to individual patients. You can refuse to participate in the most blatant forms of discrimination. What you can't change, is the fact that Medicaid reimbursement is lower than private insurance, which creates financial incentives for healthcare systems to invest more resources in predominantly White patient populations. You can't change that Black and Brown patients are more likely to be uninsured or underinsured, limiting their access to comprehensive care.

Healthcare workers become complicit in racist care structures simply by working within them. They can't opt out—they need employment, they have student loans, they have to work somewhere, but working within structurally racist healthcare systems means participating in those systems' perpetuation of racial health inequities, even while trying to provide the best care possible to individual patients.

This is moral injury specific to healthcare's racial hierarchies: being forced to participate in systems that harm patients based on race, seeing those harms clearly, and being unable to prevent them because the inequities are built into the fundamental structure of American healthcare financing and delivery.

Why Providers Don't Quit: The Golden Handcuffs

Given the suffering, the moral injury, and the systematic destruction of healthcare workers' well-being, the question arises: why don't they all quit?

Some do. Most stay, though, trapped by what's commonly called the "golden handcuffs"—financial obligations that make leaving impossible despite the psychological cost of staying.

Medical school debt is the primary mechanism. The average medical school graduate carries hundreds of thousands of dollars in student loan debt. Many owe $300,000 to $500,000 by the time they finish training. These are not normal student loans. They're massive financial obligations requiring physician-level salaries to service.

Monthly loan payments can easily exceed $3,000 to $4,000. Over a standard repayment period, physicians pay hundreds of thousands in interest on top of the original principal. The debt load requires continuous employment at high salaries. Taking time off isn't an option. Reducing hours isn't feasible. Working in lower-paid settings becomes financially impossible.

This means physicians suffering severe burnout and moral injury can't leave clinical practice without defaulting on loans. They're financially trapped in jobs that are destroying them psychologically. The system uses debt to ensure compliance. You can't walk away when leaving means financial catastrophe.

The debt trap is deliberate. Medical education could be publicly funded, as it is in many countries. Instead, the United States forces physicians to take on crushing debt loads, ensuring they'll be financially dependent on physician salaries for decades after graduation. This creates a workforce that must continue working regardless of the conditions, because the alternative is bankruptcy.

Health insurance ties workers further to employment. Losing your job means losing health coverage for yourself and your family. In a country where healthcare costs can be catastrophic, losing insurance is a risk many people can't take. Healthcare workers stay in harmful jobs because their families depend on the health coverage that employment provides.

The irony is brutal: healthcare workers are trapped in jobs that destroy their health because leaving would cost them their health insurance. The system that creates their suffering also ensures they can't escape it.

Supporting families adds additional pressure. Many healthcare workers are primary earners for their households. They have mortgages, children's education to fund, elderly parents to help support. The financial obligations extend beyond personal debt to family responsibilities that require stable, high income.

Walking away from medicine means walking away from the salary needed to meet all these obligations. Some can make that choice. Many can't. They're trapped between psychological destruction from staying and financial destruction from leaving.

I took a two-year hiatus from full-time clinical practice after COVID. The work had become unbearable—not just the pandemic stress, but the underlying conditions that COVID made worse. The expectation to see patient after patient with inadequate time. The back-to-back patient visits with no breaks. The constant time pressure. The knowing you're providing superficial care because deep care requires time the system doesn't allocate.

I could take that hiatus because I'm a locums provider—contract work, not permanent employment, which gives me more flexibility than most providers have. Even so, stepping away meant giving up income, accepting financial uncertainty, and dealing with the fear that comes from not having stable employment in a system that demands continuous work to service debt and maintain living standards.

Most providers can't take that time away. They have permanent positions, established practices, partnership tracks that would be derailed by leaving. They have student loans requiring monthly payments regardless of whether they're working. They have families depending on their income and health insurance. They're financially handcuffed to positions that are destroying them.

The system counts on this. It creates conditions that would drive anyone away, then makes leaving financially impossible. The debt ensures compliance. The insurance dependence ensures continued work. The family obligations ensure staying in harmful jobs because the alternative is harming the people you're responsible for supporting.

This is how American healthcare maintains a workforce despite treating that workforce brutally. It traps people with debt, with insurance dependence, with financial obligations that require continued high-income employment. It makes leaving more damaging than staying, even when staying is causing profound psychological harm.

The golden handcuffs are structural, not individual. You can't escape through better financial planning or more frugal living. The debt loads are too large. The income requirements are too high. The insurance dependence is too critical. The system is designed to trap healthcare workers in employment regardless of the cost to their psychological and physical health.

This serves institutional interests perfectly. Healthcare corporations and insurance companies benefit from having a workforce that can't leave despite terrible working conditions. They can impose productivity requirements, deny clinical autonomy, force participation in harmful practices, and pay providers less than the value they generate—all while knowing the workforce is trapped and can't quit en masse no matter how bad conditions become.

The moral injury is compounded by this trap. Healthcare workers aren't just forced to participate in harmful systems—they're financially prevented from escaping those systems. They watch themselves being destroyed, understand what's happening, and continue anyway because debt and family obligations leave no alternative. The awareness that you're trapped increases the psychological damage of the trap itself.

The System Working As Designed

Provider burnout and moral injury aren't bugs in American healthcare. They're features. The system creates these conditions deliberately and maintains them because they serve institutional interests.

Exhausted, burned out, morally injured healthcare workers are less likely to organize for systemic change. They're too depleted to fight.

They're focused on surviving each day rather than on transforming the conditions making survival so difficult. Burnout keeps healthcare workers politically demobilized, which protects the profitable status quo.

Moral injury serves similar functions. Healthcare workers who feel complicit in harm, who blame themselves for systemic failures, who experience shame about the inadequate care they're forced to provide—these workers don't organize effectively. They're too busy managing their own guilt and psychological damage to build movements for change.

The system benefits from this. If healthcare workers united to demand adequate staffing, reasonable schedules, time to provide proper care, freedom from insurance company interference, and structural changes to prioritize patients over profit—they could force significant reforms. The healthcare workforce has enormous leverage. Without physicians, nurses, and other healthcare workers, the system cannot function. If they collectively refused to work under current conditions, the system would have to change.

It's just that collective action requires energy, hope, and solidarity. Burnout depletes energy. Moral injury destroys hope. The golden handcuffs prevent solidarity by making each worker too focused on individual financial survival to risk their employment through collective action.

Breaking healthcare workers maintains profitable dysfunction. As long as the workforce stays broken—too exhausted to organize, too morally injured to believe change is possible, too financially trapped to leave—the system can continue extracting maximum profit while providing minimum care.

The corporate response to burnout reveals this clearly. Healthcare institutions respond to workforce suffering with "wellness programs" and "resilience training." They offer yoga classes, meditation apps, and seminars on stress management. They locate the problem in individual providers' inability to cope rather than in the systemic conditions creating the suffering.

This framing is deliberate. If burnout results from individual weakness or poor coping skills, the solution is teaching individuals to tolerate intolerable conditions better. If burnout results from systemic exploitation, the solution is changing the system—which would reduce profits.

So the system offers resilience training instead of reasonable work hours. It provides wellness programs instead of adequate staffing. It teaches stress management instead of eliminating the insurance denials and corporate policies creating the stress. This approach guarantees that conditions don't improve while making it appear that institutions are addressing the problem.

Some changes do help. Reducing work hours decreases burnout—which reveals that overwork is a cause. Adding scribes and clerical support improves provider well-being—which reveals that administrative burden is a cause. These interventions prove that systemic factors create burnout, yet healthcare institutions resist systemic changes because those changes would reduce productivity and profit.

The consequences of provider burnout extend beyond individual suffering to affect patient care quality. Burned out healthcare workers make more errors. Patient safety incidents double when providers are burned out. Low professionalism doubles. Patient dissatisfaction doubles. The system's destruction of its workforce directly harms patients.

The system fully accepts this. Medical errors, patient safety incidents, and dissatisfaction are costs the system is willing to bear in exchange for maintaining high productivity and profit margins. Reducing burnout would require reducing patient volume, increasing staffing, allowing more time per patient—all of which would reduce revenue. The system chooses revenue over both healthcare worker wellbeing and patient safety.

This is the fundamental truth: American healthcare destroys its workforce intentionally, systematically, and profitably. The burnout and moral injury aren't unfortunate side effects of a system trying its best under difficult circumstances. They're predictable outcomes of a system designed to extract maximum labor from healthcare workers at minimum cost while making them complicit in harm they can recognize but can't prevent.

The suffering serves the system. The demoralization serves the system. The financial traps serve the system. The weaponization of providers against patients serves the system. The moral injury that makes healthcare workers feel like failures rather than recognizing themselves as exploited workers within an exploitative system—that serves the system most of all.

As long as healthcare workers stay broken, stay trapped, stay convinced that their suffering is personal failure rather than systemic exploitation—the system continues unchanged. The profits continue flowing, the harm continues accumulating, and another generation of healthcare workers enters the field with idealism and hope, only to be systematically destroyed by a system designed to consume them.

The burnout and moral injury aren't problems the system is trying to solve. They're mechanisms the system uses to maintain control, suppress resistance, and ensure that the people who understand the system's cruelty most intimately are too damaged to effectively fight it.

This is fundamental for the predatory system we're all victims of. It was never designed to prevent these outcomes, and now it requires us to react against them.

> *First, though, we must understand the difference between prevention and reaction to not repeat falling victims to a profit-based system ever again.*

PART 4

WHAT WE DESERVE

CHAPTER

11 Preventive VS. Reactive

The Woman Who Couldn't Get Preventive Care

The following scenario is a composite constructed from patterns documented in American healthcare. The details are hypothetical, but the dynamics are widespread and common.

Janet Morrison was 52 years old when her doctor told her she was headed for a heart attack. Not today, not tomorrow, but inevitably if nothing changed. Her blood pressure was creeping up—not high enough for medication yet, just high enough to worry about. Her cholesterol was borderline. Her father had died of a heart attack at 58. Her brother had bypass surgery at 55. The warning signs were clear, documented, and undeniable.

Her doctor recommended what the evidence says works: dietary counseling with a registered nutritionist, a structured exercise program, stress management techniques, and close monitoring. Catch the problems now, before they become disease. Prevent the heart attack rather than treating it after the damage is done.

Her insurance company said no. Not covered. Not medically necessary. She didn't have heart disease yet, so prevention wasn't justified. Come back when you've had a heart attack, then we'll pay for treatment.

The nutritionist charged $200 per session. Janet would need at least six sessions to develop a sustainable plan. That's $1,200 out-of-pocket—money she didn't have. The exercise program her doctor recommended cost $150 monthly. Another $1,800 annually. The stress management counseling wasn't covered either. She was looking at $3,000-4,000 in preventive care costs that insurance refused to cover because she wasn't sick enough yet.

So she did what millions of Americans do: nothing. She couldn't afford the prevention her doctor recommended. She hoped her genetics wouldn't catch up to her. She tried to eat better and exercise more on her own, without professional guidance, without structured support, without the interventions proven to prevent what was coming.

Five years later, at 57, Janet Morrison had a massive heart attack. She survived—barely. Three days in cardiac ICU. Emergency angioplasty. Two stents placed in blocked arteries. A week in the hospital. Cardiac rehabilitation after discharge. A lifetime of medications. Permanent heart damage that would limit her activity and require ongoing monitoring for the rest of her life.

The hospital bill exceeded $150,000. Insurance paid it. Every penny of the acute crisis care that could have been prevented for $3,000 five years earlier.

This isn't system failure. This is system design.

The insurance company made a calculated decision: refuse to pay $3,000 for prevention that would keep Janet healthy, wait for the inevitable crisis, then pay $150,000 for treatment. Why? Because the $150,000 came from premiums collected across millions of policy holders, while the $3,000 would have been a direct cost. Because prevention doesn't generate revenue for hospitals, pharmaceutical companies, or medical device manufacturers. Because, as outlined in earlier chapters, keeping Janet healthy would mean she didn't need expensive cardiac care, and expensive cardiac care is where the money is.

Janet's heart attack generated revenue for everyone in the healthcare system except Janet. The hospital billed $150,000. The cardiologist billed $8,000. The pharmaceutical companies will collect thousands annually for the medications she'll take for life. The insurance company collected her premiums for five years without paying out for prevention, then paid for treatment knowing they'd recoup costs through higher premiums charged to everyone.

The only person who lost was Janet—permanently damaged heart, reduced quality of life, constant medication regimen, fear of the next cardiac event. Her suffering was profitable—her prevention would not have been.

This is American healthcare: designed to maximize treatment revenue, not health.

Why Prevention Doesn't Pay

As you have been shown, the American healthcare system doesn't profit from keeping people healthy. It profits from treating sick people. This isn't a controversial statement—it's the fundamental business model.

Hospitals make money from procedures, surgeries, and hospitalizations. Empty beds don't generate revenue. Preventing hospitalizations means losing income. Every patient who doesn't need emergency surgery is money not earned. Every heart attack prevented is tens of thousands in lost billing. Every cancer caught so early it requires only minimal treatment is revenue that never materializes.

The financial incentive is explicit: keep beds full, keep operating rooms busy, keep emergency departments crowded. Prevention empties beds. Prevention reduces procedures. Prevention cuts into hospital revenue. Why would hospitals invest in prevention that directly reduces their income?

Pharmaceutical companies profit from medications for chronic disease. Diabetes generates billions in insulin sales. High blood pressure generates billions in antihypertensive medication sales. High cholesterol generates billions in statin sales. Depression generates billions in antidepressant sales. These are profitable conditions precisely because they require lifelong medication.

Preventing diabetes means no insulin sales.

Preventing hypertension means no blood pressure medication sales.

Preventing the conditions that require pharmaceutical intervention means eliminating revenue streams worth billions annually.

Why would pharmaceutical companies support prevention that eliminates their markets?

Insurance companies profit from premiums collected minus claims paid. Prevention requires upfront investment—paying for nutritionist visits, exercise programs, mental health counseling, regular screenings, early interventions. These costs are immediate and direct. The benefits—fewer hospitalizations, less chronic disease, lower treatment costs—accrue over years or decades.

But patients change insurance companies. They switch jobs. They age into Medicare. They move between employer plans, marketplace plans, and Medicaid. The insurance company that pays for prevention today likely won't be the insurer collecting the cost savings five or ten years later when that prevention prevents expensive acute care.

Why invest in prevention when another insurer will reap the savings? Better to minimize preventive care spending and compete on premium costs today. Let future insurers—or Medicare—deal with the expensive consequences of prevention avoided.

Providers are paid fee-for-service—for the volume of patients seen and procedures performed, not for health outcomes. A primary care provider who spends 45 minutes counseling a patient on lifestyle changes to prevent diabetes gets paid for one visit. A specialist who performs a procedure gets paid substantially more. The economic incentives favor procedures over prevention, specialists over primary care, treatment over counseling.

A cardiologist performing an angioplasty makes thousands. A primary care physician preventing the heart attack that would have required angioplasty makes a fraction of that through routine office visits spread over years. The prevention is more valuable to the patient and society—but less profitable to the provider.

Every major player in American healthcare loses revenue if the system shifts to prevention:

- Hospitals lose revenue from prevented hospitalizations
- Pharmaceutical companies lose revenue from preventing chronic disease
- Specialists lose revenue from prevented acute care interventions
- Insurance companies invest in prevention but other insurers collect the savings
- Medical device manufacturers lose revenue from prevented procedures

The only entities that benefit from prevention are patients (who stay healthier) and society (which pays less overall). But patients and society don't control the healthcare system. The entities that profit from illness do.

This is why prevention doesn't happen despite overwhelming evidence that it works better and costs less. The evidence doesn't matter. The financial incentives are completely backward. The system is optimized for revenue generation, not health. Keeping people healthy reduces income across the healthcare industry, while making people healthy after they get sick generates maximum revenue.

Prevention requires investment with delayed returns. Treatment generates immediate revenue. The system chooses revenue every single time.

This isn't conspiracy. It's basic economics. When profit depends on treating illness, prevention becomes a threat to the business model. The system responds rationally to its incentive structure—by avoiding prevention and focusing on treatment.

Janet Morrison's heart attack was good for the healthcare system's bottom line. Her prevention would not have been. That's why she was denied preventive care and given excellent acute care after her heart attack. The system worked exactly as designed: maximize treatment revenue by avoiding prevention.

What Reactive Healthcare Looks Like

American healthcare excels in crisis. If you're having a heart attack, there's no better place in the world to be than a U.S. emergency room. Trauma care, emergency surgery, acute interventions—the United States is world-class at treating medical emergencies. We're exceptional at saving people who are actively dying.

We're terrible at keeping people from getting sick in the first place.

This reactive approach permeates the entire system. We wait for illness to develop, progress, become serious, and then deploy expensive interventions. We treat symptoms after they appear rather than addressing risk factors before disease develops. We excel at rescuing people from medical crises we could have prevented.

Heart disease is the leading cause of death in America. We have the world's most advanced cardiac care—angioplasty, bypass surgery, stents, pacemakers, heart transplants. We can keep hearts beating through extraordinary interventions. We're terrible at preventing the heart disease that requires these interventions.

Other countries prevent heart disease through blood pressure management, cholesterol control, dietary counseling, exercise promotion, and smoking cessation—all provided at little or no cost to patients. These countries have far lower rates of cardiac events requiring acute intervention.

The United States waits until people have heart attacks, then provides world-class treatment. We're better at fixing broken hearts than preventing them from breaking.

Cancer treatment in the U.S. is cutting-edge. Chemotherapy, radiation, targeted therapies, immunotherapy, surgical oncology—we have the most advanced cancer treatment in the world. We're substantially worse at cancer prevention and early detection.

Countries with universal healthcare provide comprehensive cancer screening at no cost. Mammograms, colonoscopies, cervical cancer screening, lung cancer screening for high-risk patients—all free at point of care, provided proactively to catch cancer early when it's most treatable.

The U.S. makes screening contingent on insurance coverage, requires prior authorization, charges patients deductibles and coinsurance, and creates barriers that delay screening until cancer is advanced. Then we deploy expensive treatment for disease that could have been caught early or prevented.

We're excellent at treating advanced cancer. We're mediocre at preventing it or catching it early.

Diabetes in America generates tens of billions in pharmaceutical revenue annually. Insulin, test strips, glucose monitors, medications for diabetes complications—it's an enormous market. We're excellent at managing diabetes with medications and technology.

We're terrible at preventing Type 2 diabetes despite clear evidence that lifestyle interventions work. Diabetes prevention programs reduce diabetes incidence by 58% in high-risk individuals. These programs cost $300-500 per person. They're rarely covered by insurance because they're "preventive."

Instead, we wait for people to develop diabetes, then spend thousands annually on medications and management for the rest of their lives. A disease that could be prevented for $500 becomes a lifetime cost of $100,000+. This is profitable for pharmaceutical companies and healthcare systems. It's devastating for patients.

Emergency rooms across America are full of preventable conditions. Hypertension that should have been managed with medication and lifestyle changes before it caused stroke. Diabetes complications that could have been prevented with early intervention and disease management. Asthma attacks that could have been avoided with controller medications and trigger avoidance. Infections that could have been stopped with timely treatment before they became sepsis.

The people in emergency rooms aren't there because medicine failed. They're there because prevention failed—or more accurately, because prevention was never provided. They couldn't afford primary care. Their insurance wouldn't cover preventive medications. They couldn't get appointments for non-emergency problems. They waited until symptoms became unbearable because seeking care earlier was unaffordable or inaccessible.

The emergency room visit costs $5,000-10,000. The preventive primary care that could have avoided it costs $200-500. Insurance pays for the emergency room. It often doesn't pay for the prevention.

This is reactive healthcare: wait for crisis, deploy expensive intervention, generate maximum revenue, and repeat. It's the opposite of what evidence says works. But it's what the system incentivizes.

The United States is the best place in the world to have a medical emergency. It's one of the worst places in the developed world to stay healthy and avoid medical emergencies in the first place.

That's not an accident. That's design. Reactive care is profitable. Preventive care is not. The system optimizes for profit.

The Cost of Reactive Care

The United States spent $14,775 per capita on healthcare in 2024—nearly double the mean of $7,860 for comparable developed nations including Australia, Austria, Belgium, Canada, France, Germany, Japan, Netherlands, Sweden, Switzerland, and the United Kingdom. We spent 1.88 times more per person than peer countries while achieving substantially worse health outcomes.

In 2024, the U.S. spent 17.2% of GDP on healthcare—more than 50% higher than comparable countries, which averaged 11.2% of GDP. We dedicate more than one-sixth of our entire economy to healthcare while other wealthy nations accomplish better health outcomes spending about half as much per capita.

Switzerland, the highest spender among peer nations after the U.S., spent approximately $9,775 per capita—still $5,000 less than the United States. Other peer nations spend even less, averaging $7,860 per capita.

For this extraordinary spending, Americans get:

Life expectancy of 78.8 years—the lowest among 11 high-income countries. Other nations ranged from 80.7 to 83.9 years, with a mean of 81.7 years. Americans die, on average, three years earlier than citizens of peer nations despite spending nearly twice as much on healthcare ($14,775 vs. $7,860 average).

Infant mortality of 5.8 deaths per 1,000 live births—the highest among developed nations. The mean for comparable countries was 3.6 per 1,000. American babies die at rates 60% higher than peer nations.

The highest obesity rate at 70.1% of adults overweight or obese—compared to a range of 23.8% to 63.4% in other nations, with a mean of 55.6%. Only America has more than two-thirds of its adult population overweight or obese.

We're spending more and getting less. Substantially less. Americans live shorter lives, babies die more frequently, chronic disease rates are higher, and health outcomes across virtually every metric are worse than peer nations spending half as much.

Why?

Because other countries invest in prevention. They catch disease early when it's cheap to treat. They manage chronic conditions to prevent complications. They provide preventive care at little or no cost to patients, removing financial barriers to early intervention. They keep people healthy rather than waiting for them to get sick.

The United States waits for crisis, then deploys expensive interventions. This costs more and achieves worse outcomes. The spending gap between the U.S. and other countries varies by age, but it's substantial across all age groups: for adults aged 20-64, U.S. spending was 2.3-fold higher; for those 65 and older, it was 2.0-fold higher. In absolute dollars, the gap peaked at $18,645 for ages 80-84—the United States was spending nearly $19,000 more per elderly person annually than comparable nations.

That additional spending didn't buy better outcomes. Even privileged white U.S. citizens in the highest-income counties had worse health outcomes than average residents of other developed countries. The U.S. health disadvantage extends across socioeconomic levels—even our wealthiest, most privileged citizens have worse health than middle-class citizens in peer nations.

The spending difference isn't driven by Americans using more healthcare. Utilization rates are largely similar across countries. Americans don't go to doctors more often, don't get more procedures, and don't stay in hospitals longer. The difference is price.

Administrative costs in the U.S. account for 8% of healthcare spending versus 1-3% in other countries. Pharmaceutical spending in the U.S. is $1,443 per capita versus $466-939 in other countries. Total per capita spending in the U.S. reached $14,775 in 2024 compared to a peer country average of $7,860. Americans pay dramatically more for the same medications, the same procedures, the same care.

The higher costs reflect pricing failure, not overuse. We're being charged far more for healthcare than citizens of other developed nations, and we're getting far less health in return.

Reactive care is expensive. Treating heart attacks costs $150,000. Preventing them costs $2,000-5,000. Treating advanced cancer costs

$200,000-500,000. Catching it early costs $5,000-20,000. Managing diabetes complications costs $100,000+ over a lifetime. Preventing diabetes costs $500.

The math is overwhelming: prevention is vastly cheaper than reactive treatment. Every dollar spent on prevention saves $3-10 in treatment costs. This isn't controversial. It's documented, researched, proven.

We're not spending more because we don't know better. We're spending more because the system profits from expensive reactive care. Prevention would save money—but savings accrue to patients and society, not to hospitals, pharmaceutical companies, and specialists who profit from treating advanced disease.

The United States is spending itself into an economic catastrophe on healthcare that delivers worse outcomes than peer nations spending half as much. This isn't because American medicine is less advanced—our acute care is world-class. It's because the system is designed to maximize treatment revenue rather than health.

We could spend less and achieve better outcomes by shifting to prevention. Every other developed nation has proven this works. We refuse because reactive care, despite costing twice as much and achieving worse results, is more profitable for the healthcare industry.

Americans are paying with their wallets, their health, and their lives for a system designed to generate revenue rather than health.

What Preventive Healthcare Looks Like

Preventive healthcare is simple in concept: catch problems early when they're cheap and easy to fix. Address risk factors before they become disease. Support healthy behaviors that prevent illness. Manage chronic conditions to prevent complications. Keep people healthy rather than waiting for them to get sick.

Other developed nations have built healthcare systems around this principle. They provide comprehensive preventive services at little or no cost to patients, removing financial barriers to early intervention. They emphasize primary care over specialist care. They invest in public health alongside medical care. They measure success by population health outcomes, not treatment revenue.

In countries with universal healthcare, preventive care is free at point of service. Annual health checks, cancer screenings, immunizations, blood pressure monitoring, cholesterol testing, diabetes screening—all provided without cost to patients. No copays, no deductibles, no prior authorization requirements, no insurance denials.

The logic is straightforward: if the goal is keeping people healthy, you remove barriers to preventive care. Financial barriers are the most significant—people avoid care they can't afford. Universal healthcare eliminates cost as a barrier to prevention.

Nutrition counseling and dietary support are covered when medically indicated. If a patient is pre-diabetic, at risk for heart disease, or has other conditions improved by dietary changes, they receive professional nutritionist services. Exercise programs for patients with chronic conditions are covered. Smoking cessation programs are free or very low cost. Mental health services—counseling, therapy, and psychiatric care—are accessible without prohibitive costs.

The investment in prevention is understood as investment in avoiding future treatment costs. Countries with universal healthcare aren't being generous—they're being economically rational. Spending $500 on diabetes prevention saves $100,000 in lifetime diabetes treatment costs. Spending $2,000 on cardiac risk management saves $150,000 in heart attack treatment. The return on investment (ROI) is obvious, and universal healthcare systems capture that return because patients don't switch insurers.

Primary care is the foundation of preventive healthcare systems. Most countries have more primary care physicians than specialists, while the U.S. is specialist-dominant. In universal healthcare systems, patients have ongoing relationships with primary care providers who know their history, manage chronic conditions, coordinate care across specialties, and provide preventive counseling over years or decades.

That continuity enables prevention. Your primary care doctor knows your family history, your risk factors, your previous conditions, your medications, your lifestyle. They can identify problems early because they're monitoring you regularly. They can intervene before disease develops because they're seeing patterns across years, not just addressing acute symptoms in isolated encounters.

In the U.S., patients often lack consistent primary care. They see different providers at urgent care clinics. They access care episodically when symptoms are too severe to ignore. They don't have doctors who know them well enough to catch problems early. The fragmented, reactive system prevents the ongoing relationships that enable prevention.

Countries with universal healthcare also invest in community health workers—non-physician providers who support patients with chronic conditions, help navigate healthcare systems, provide education, and offer ongoing monitoring and support. These workers keep people engaged with preventive care, ensure medication adherence, identify problems early, and provide the kind of sustained support that prevents complications.

Home visits for elderly patients, pregnant women, and people with chronic conditions are common in many universal healthcare systems. Providers go to patients rather than waiting for patients to come in when problems are severe. This enables early intervention, medication management, lifestyle support, and identification of problems before they require hospitalization.

Mental health care is integrated with medical care rather than separated and poorly covered. Depression screening, anxiety treatment, substance abuse support—these are part of comprehensive healthcare, not add-ons that patients can't afford. The integration reflects understanding that mental health and physical health are inseparable, and that untreated mental health conditions lead to worse physical health outcomes.

Dental and vision care are covered, not separated as they are in the U.S. This matters because dental disease and vision problems have systemic health effects. Untreated dental infections cause heart disease. Vision problems lead to falls and injuries. Treating the whole person rather than fragmenting care by body system enables better prevention.

The measurement of success is different. Universal healthcare systems track population health outcomes—life expectancy, infant mortality, disease rates, and disability rates. They're incentivized to keep populations healthy because the system bears the cost of illness. Preventive care that reduces future treatment needs is directly beneficial to the system.

In the U.S., success is measured by revenue, patient volume, and procedure counts. Hospitals track bed occupancy rates. Physicians track relative value units (RVUs) measuring billable activities. Insurance companies track medical loss ratios—the percentage of premiums paid out for care, with lower ratios meaning higher profits. None of these metrics incentivize prevention. All incentivize maximizing treatment volume.

Preventive healthcare looks fundamentally different from what most Americans experience. It's proactive rather than reactive. It's continuous rather than episodic. It's coordinated rather than fragmented. It's focused on health outcomes rather than billable procedures. It removes financial barriers rather than creating them. It keeps people healthy rather than waiting for them to get sick.

Most importantly: it works. Countries that have built healthcare systems around prevention spend half as much as the United States while achieving substantially better health outcomes. The model exists. It's proven.

We're not applying it because it's less profitable than reactive care.

International Comparisons: Outcomes

Every other developed nation achieves better health outcomes than the United States despite spending far less. This isn't close. It's not a statistical tie. American health outcomes are consistently, measurably, substantially worse than peer nations across virtually every metric.

Life expectancy: Americans live 78.8 years on average—the lowest among 11 high-income countries. Japan's life expectancy is 83.9 years. Switzerland is 83.4 years. Australia, Canada, France, Germany, Netherlands, Norway, Sweden, and the UK all exceed 80 years. The mean life expectancy for comparator nations is 81.7 years—nearly three years longer than Americans live.

Three years. That's not a rounding error. That's the entire difference between a system designed to keep people healthy and a system designed to treat sick people. Americans die years earlier than citizens of peer nations while spending twice as much on healthcare.

The life expectancy gap appears early and persists across the lifespan. American infant mortality is higher. American children have higher rates of preventable death. American adults develop chronic disease earlier and die from it at higher rates. American elderly face higher rates of disability and complications from poorly managed chronic conditions.

Even White Americans in the highest-income counties—the most advantaged population in the United States—have worse health outcomes than average residents of other developed countries. The U.S. health disadvantage isn't explained by poverty, lack of education, or poor health behaviors among disadvantaged populations. Even our wealthiest, most privileged citizens are less healthy than middle-class citizens of peer nations.

Infant mortality: The United States has 5.8 deaths per 1,000 live births—the highest rate among developed nations. The mean for comparable countries is 3.6 per 1,000. American babies die at rates 60% higher than babies in peer nations.

Japan has an infant mortality rate of 1.8 per 1,000—meaning

Japanese babies are more than three times as likely to survive their first year than American babies. Nordic countries have rates around 2-3 per 1,000. France, Germany, UK, Canada, Australia—all substantially lower than the United States.

This isn't because American medicine can't save sick babies. Our neonatal intensive care is world-class. The problem is prevention: inadequate prenatal care, poor maternal health, lack of support for pregnant women, and births that are preventably premature or complicated.

Other countries provide comprehensive prenatal care at no cost. Regular checkups, nutrition support, risk screening, and early intervention for complications. They keep pregnant women healthy, preventing premature births and complications that require NICU care. They invest in prevention and see infant mortality drop dramatically as a result.

The United States charges for prenatal care, creates barriers to access, provides inadequate support for pregnant women, and then deploys excellent neonatal intensive care when babies are born too early or too sick. We're reactive when prevention would save lives and cost less.

Maternal mortality: The United States has approximately 32.9 deaths per 100,000 live births—the highest rate in the developed world and getting worse. Most European countries have maternal mortality rates below 10 per 100,000. The U.S. rate is three to four times higher than peer nations.

American women are dying from preventable pregnancy-related complications at rates unseen in any other wealthy nation. These deaths are concentrated among Black women, who face maternal mortality rates three to four times higher than White women—approaching rates seen in developing nations rather than developed ones.

Other countries provide comprehensive maternal care throughout pregnancy and postpartum. Regular monitoring, management of chronic conditions, treatment of complications, postpartum support. They prevent the hemorrhages, infections, blood pressure crises, and other complications that kill American women.

The United States provides fragmented prenatal care contingent on insurance coverage, inadequate postpartum support, and poor management of conditions like hypertension and diabetes during pregnancy. We're excellent at emergency obstetric interventions when women are dying. We're terrible at preventing those emergencies.

Chronic disease: The United States has 70.1% of adults overweight or obese—the highest rate among developed nations. Other countries range from 23.8% to 63.4%, with a mean of 55.6%. Only America has more than two-thirds of adults overweight or obese.

This isn't coincidental. America's food regulatory system—which allows ingredients that are banned in Europe because they're linked to obesity, metabolic disease, and cancer—creates the chronic conditions that healthcare then profits from treating. I examine this connected crisis in my forthcoming book, *Poisoned For Profit: The Food That's Killing Americans (And Why the FDA Allows It).*

Obesity drives diabetes, heart disease, stroke, certain cancers, and numerous other conditions. Countries with lower obesity rates achieve this through public health interventions, nutrition programs, walkable urban design, food policy, and healthcare systems that support weight management.

The United States has higher rates of diabetes, hypertension, and cardiovascular disease than peer nations. These are largely preventable conditions—manageable through lifestyle, diet, exercise, early intervention, and ongoing medical management. Other countries prevent or manage these conditions better, resulting in lower rates of complications and better health outcomes.

The outcomes gap is comprehensive. Americans have higher rates of virtually every chronic disease. We develop these conditions earlier in life. We manage them less effectively. We experience more complications. We die from them at higher rates.

This isn't because American medicine is less advanced. Our treatment of acute complications from chronic disease is world-class. But we're terrible at prevention, early detection, and ongoing management—the approaches that other countries use to keep people healthier.

Quality of care: Even when controlling for the higher disease burden in the U.S., quality metrics show comparable or worse performance than peer nations. Rates of preventable hospitalizations, medical errors, healthcare-associated infections, and adverse events are similar to or higher than other countries.

We're not getting better quality care to justify the higher costs. We're getting similar or worse quality while paying twice as much. The spending difference goes to administrative costs, pharmaceutical profits, and higher prices for everything—not to better care.

The international comparisons are damning. Every developed nation achieves better health outcomes spending far less. They do this through universal coverage that removes financial barriers, emphasis on primary care and prevention, coordination of care, and healthcare systems designed to optimize health rather than revenue.

The United States could achieve better outcomes at lower cost by adopting approaches proven successful in every peer nation. We don't because reactive care, despite being more expensive and less effective, is more profitable for the healthcare industry.

Americans are living shorter, sicker lives than citizens of peer nations. This isn't inevitable. It's a policy choice. We're choosing profit over health, and people are dying as a result.

International Comparisons: Costs

The United States spent $14,775 per capita on healthcare in 2024—nearly double comparable nations. This spending gap is consistent, enormous, and unjustifiable given the worse outcomes Americans experience. Healthcare spending grew 7.5% in 2023 alone—outpacing GDP growth for the first time since the pandemic.

Let's break down what other countries spend:

United Kingdom: $6,747 per capita (less than half U.S. spending). The NHS provides comprehensive healthcare to all residents. No premiums, no deductibles, no copays for most services. Preventive care is emphasized. Primary care is the foundation. Life expectancy exceeds the U.S. by more than two years.

Japan: $5,790 per capita (less than half U.S. spending). Universal coverage through statutory insurance. Life expectancy of 83.9

years—five years longer than Americans. Infant mortality of 1.8 per 1,000—less than one-third the U.S. rate. The world's longest-living population, achieved at about 40% of U.S. cost.

Canada: $7,301 per capita (about half U.S. spending). Universal single-payer system (Medicare for All, actually implemented). All medically necessary care covered. No medical bankruptcies. Life expectancy exceeds the U.S. by three years. Infant mortality is substantially lower.

France: $7,367 per capita (about half U.S. spending). Universal multi-payer system with strong regulation. Consistently ranks among the world's best healthcare systems. Better outcomes across virtually all metrics. Half the cost.

Germany: $9,365 per capita (still $5,410 less than U.S. spending). Universal statutory health insurance. Comprehensive coverage. Better health outcomes at substantially lower costs.

Switzerland: $9,963 per capita—the highest spender among peer nations, still $4,812 less than the United States. Universal coverage. Better outcomes. Still dramatically cheaper.

Australia: $7,469 per capita (about half U.S. spending). Universal Medicare system supplemented by private insurance. Comprehensive coverage. Better outcomes at about half the cost.

The pattern is consistent: every developed nation spends dramatically less than the United States while achieving better health outcomes. The spending gap ranges from 1.7-fold to 2.5-fold—meaning Americans pay approximately two times more per person for healthcare that delivers worse results.

In 2024, the U.S. spent 17.2% of GDP on healthcare—more than one-sixth of the entire economy. Comparable countries averaged 11.2% of GDP. The U.S. dedicates more than 50% additional economic resources to healthcare while achieving inferior outcomes.

This isn't close. It's not a marginal difference. The spending gap represents nearly $6,915 per person annually ($14,775 - $7,860). That's money Americans are spending on healthcare that could be saved while achieving better outcomes if we adopted approaches used in every other peer nation.

Where does the extra money go? Not to better care—outcomes are worse. Not to more utilization—Americans don't use substantially more healthcare services. The money goes to:

Administrative costs: 8% of U.S. healthcare spending versus 1-3% in other countries. The complexity of American insurance—multiple payers, prior authorization, billing disputes, denial appeals, coordination across fragmented systems—generates massive administrative overhead that contributes nothing to health.

Pharmaceutical costs: $1,443 per capita in the U.S. versus $466-939 in other countries. Americans pay two to three times more for identical medications. Other countries negotiate drug prices nationally. The U.S. prohibits Medicare from negotiating and allows pharmaceutical companies to charge whatever they want.

Higher prices for everything: Hospital stays, procedures, specialist visits, diagnostic tests—all cost dramatically more in the United States than other countries for identical care. The pricing is not based on cost or value. It's based on market power and the ability to charge whatever insurance will pay or patients can be forced to pay.

Profit extraction: Insurance company profits, pharmaceutical profits, hospital profits, profits for private equity firms buying medical practices and hospitals. Other countries have universal non-profit systems or heavily regulated insurance markets. The U.S. allows unrestricted profit extraction from healthcare.

The spending difference doesn't buy better outcomes. It buys profit for healthcare corporations. Americans are paying nearly twice as much to generate corporate profits while receiving worse care.

The spending gap varies by age but exists across all age groups. For adults aged 20-64, U.S. spending was 2.3-fold higher than peer nations. For those 65 and older, it was 2.0-fold higher. In absolute dollars, the gap peaked at $18,645 annually for ages 80-84—the U.S. was spending nearly $19,000 more per elderly person than comparable nations.

That additional spending didn't result in better end-of-life care, better quality of life for elderly patients, or better management of chronic conditions. It went to profit extraction and administrative overhead.

The international cost comparisons prove that universal healthcare costs less than the U.S. system. Every nation that has implemented universal coverage spends about half as much per capita. They don't ration care—they provide more comprehensive coverage than most Americans have. They don't have worse quality—their outcomes are better across virtually all metrics.

They spend less because their systems are designed to optimize health, not profit. They emphasize prevention, coordinate care, remove administrative complexity, negotiate prices, and operate non-profit insurance systems. They don't have insurance companies denying claims to maximize profits. They don't have pharmaceutical companies charging whatever they want. They don't have hospitals billing $10,000 for procedures that cost $1,000 to provide.

The United States could cut healthcare spending in nearly in half and achieve better outcomes by adopting approaches proven successful in every peer nation. We could cover everyone, eliminate medical bankruptcy, improve health outcomes, and save trillions of dollars.

We don't because the current system is too profitable for insurance companies, pharmaceutical companies, hospitals, and private equity firms extracting wealth from healthcare. They profit from high costs. They lobby to prevent reform. They fight any change that would reduce their profits even if it would improve care and cut costs.

Americans are paying twice as much as citizens of peer nations for worse healthcare because the system is designed to maximize profit, not health. The international comparisons prove this conclusively. Better healthcare at lower cost is possible—every other developed nation has it. We're choosing not to have it because profit is prioritized over people.

The ROI of Prevention: What Research Shows

The return on investment for preventive care isn't controversial. Decades of research across multiple countries and healthcare systems consistently demonstrate that prevention saves money while improving health outcomes. Every dollar spent on prevention saves three to ten dollars in treatment costs. This is documented, proven, and overwhelmingly clear.

Yet the United States invests minimally in prevention while spending massively on reactive treatment. Why? Because the return on investment accrues to patients and society, not to the healthcare corporations that would need to invest in prevention.

Diabetes prevention: Lifestyle interventions for people at high risk of Type 2 diabetes have a median cost-effectiveness ratio of $12,510 per quality-adjusted life year (QALY)—well below the $50,000 threshold considered cost-effective. Metformin prevention has a ratio of $17,089 per QALY. The National Diabetes Prevention Program has an 88% probability of saving money over just two years.

Preventing diabetes costs $300-500 per person for a structured lifestyle intervention program. Managing diabetes costs $9,000-14,000 annually over a lifetime. The lifetime cost difference is $100,000 or more. Preventing one case of diabetes saves more than $100,000 in treatment costs while dramatically improving quality of life for the person who didn't develop a chronic disease.

Yet insurance companies routinely refuse to cover diabetes prevention programs. They're classified as "wellness" or "lifestyle" rather than medical care, making them ineligible for coverage. The person develops diabetes, then insurance pays for expensive lifetime management. Prevention would save money—but insurers don't invest because patients might switch insurance before savings materialize.

Cancer screening: Colorectal cancer screening through multi-component interventions is cost-saving, with decreases in cost per QALY of $1,651 to $3,817. This means screening doesn't just improve outcomes—it actually saves money by catching cancer early when treatment is cheaper and more effective.

HPV vaccination combined with screening has cost-effectiveness ratios ranging from $86 to $476 per QALY gained. Preventing cervical cancer through vaccination and screening is extraordinarily cost-effective—yet many insurance plans require copays for screening, create prior authorization barriers, and don't adequately cover vaccines.

Breast cancer screening, lung cancer screening for high-risk patients, and other evidence-based screening programs all show strong ROI. Catching cancer early costs less and saves more lives than treating advanced disease, but insurance often creates barriers to screening through costs, authorization requirements, and coverage limitations.

Cardiovascular disease prevention: Managing blood pressure, cholesterol, and other cardiac risk factors saves $4-8 for every dollar spent. Preventing heart attacks and strokes through medication, lifestyle support, and risk factor management is dramatically cheaper than treating cardiovascular events.

A lifetime of statins for someone with high cholesterol costs roughly $20,000-30,000. Treating a heart attack costs $150,000 initially plus ongoing care costs exceeding $100,000. Preventing the heart attack through cholesterol management saves over $200,000 while preventing death, disability, and reduced quality of life.

Yet insurers routinely deny statins for primary prevention, require "trying diet and exercise first" before covering medications, and won't cover the nutritionist or exercise program support that would make lifestyle interventions effective. They refuse to pay for prevention that would save them money.

Childhood vaccinations: The ROI on childhood vaccination programs ranges from $3 to $10 saved for every dollar spent. Vaccines prevent diseases that would require expensive treatment, cause long-term complications, and result in disability or death. The savings from preventing measles, polio, pertussis, and other vaccine-preventable diseases is enormous.

Vaccination programs are among the most cost-effective public health interventions ever implemented. They save money while dramatically improving health. Yet anti-vaccine movements have taken hold partly because the U.S. healthcare system doesn't effectively communicate the value of prevention—the system profits from treatment, not prevention.

Smoking cessation: Programs to help people quit smoking save $3-7 for every dollar spent. Smoking causes cancer, heart disease, stroke, COPD, and numerous other expensive conditions. Preventing smoking-related disease through cessation programs is extraordinarily cost-effective.

Yet insurance coverage for smoking cessation is inconsistent. Medications like varenicline (Chantix) or bupropion are often not covered or require high copays. Counseling programs are not adequately covered. The investment in cessation would pay for itself many times over—but insurers don't fully cover it.

Mental health prevention: Early intervention for depression, anxiety, and other mental health conditions prevents progression to severe mental illness, prevents substance abuse, prevents suicide, and reduces medical costs from untreated mental health conditions manifesting as physical illness.

The ROI is substantial—every dollar spent on mental health

prevention saves roughly $4 in treatment costs. Yet mental health prevention is poorly covered, if covered at all. Insurance makes accessing mental health care difficult through high copays, narrow networks, prior authorization requirements, and limited session numbers.

Maternal and prenatal care: Comprehensive prenatal care prevents premature births, complications, and maternal and infant deaths. The cost of NICU care for premature infants ranges from $50,000 to $500,000. Preventing prematurity through adequate prenatal care costs $2,000-5,000. The ROI is enormous.

Yet access to prenatal care in the U.S. is inconsistent. Many women don't have insurance when they become pregnant. Medicaid coverage varies by state. Women face barriers to accessing care early in pregnancy. The resulting premature births and complications cost vastly more than prevention would have.

The evidence is overwhelming: prevention saves money. Every major preventive intervention studied shows strong positive ROI. The United States could save hundreds of billions annually by shifting investment from reactive treatment to prevention.

We don't because the ROI accrues to patients and society, not to healthcare corporations. Insurance companies invest in prevention but other insurers collect the savings when patients switch coverage. Hospitals lose revenue from preventing hospitalizations. Pharmaceutical companies lose revenue from preventing chronic diseases. Specialists lose revenue from preventing acute events.

The financial incentives are completely backward. Everyone involved in healthcare profits from expensive treatment. Nobody profits from prevention except patients—who stay healthier—and society—which saves money. But patients and society don't control healthcare investment decisions. Corporations seeking maximum profit do.

The research proves prevention works and saves money. The system ignores that research because profit, not evidence, determines investment.

What Prevention Could Have Prevented

I've seen the consequences of denied prevention throughout my career. Not because documentation is lacking or evidence is weak, but because the system refuses to invest in prevention that would reduce treatment revenue.

Mental Health and Gun Violence:

I believe there's a direct connection between inadequate mental health access and gun violence in America. The people shooting up schools and public places are mentally ill. They're not getting treatment—not because treatment doesn't exist but because they can't access it.

Mental health care in America is terrible. Insurance doesn't adequately cover it. Copays are high. Networks are narrow. Wait times for appointments are months. People in crisis can't get help until they're so severe they require hospitalization—and even then, they're often released after 72 hours with minimal follow-up.

If Americans had access to affordable mental health care, many of these shootings wouldn't happen. Early intervention prevents crisis. Ongoing treatment prevents deterioration. Support prevents desperation.

Yet, we don't provide that care. We wait until people are actively dangerous, then we deploy crisis response. By then, people are dead. Prevention would save lives—both the victims of violence and the people who commit it because they're untreated and desperate.

This is all connected to broader healthcare dysfunction: Americans work 2-3 jobs to afford health insurance and other basic necessities. The stress, exhaustion, and financial desperation create mental health crises. People are too stressed, too broke, too exhausted to cope. They break.

If healthcare weren't tied to employment, if people didn't have to work themselves to death to afford insurance, if mental health care were accessible and affordable, we'd have fewer desperate, untreated, breaking-point people picking up guns.

The gun violence crisis and the healthcare crisis are connected. Untreated mental illness kills people. The system that denies mental health care shares responsibility for those deaths.

The Pattern: Deny Prevention, Pay for Crisis

I've watched this pattern unfold repeatedly: insurance refuses to cover prevention, patients can't afford it out-of-pocket, conditions worsen, expensive crisis occurs, insurance pays for treatment that wouldn't have been necessary if they'd covered prevention.

- It's not just the examples I've mentioned. It's everywhere:
- Patients denied physical therapy after injuries, developing chronic pain that requires surgery and long-term pain management

- Patients denied preventive cardiac medications, having heart attacks that require emergency intervention
- Patients denied mental health counseling, ending up hospitalized after suicide attempts or psychiatric crises
- Patients denied nutritionist services, developing obesity-related conditions requiring lifetime medication and management
- Patients denied early cancer screening, diagnosed at advanced stages requiring aggressive treatment

Every provider sees this. Every day. We prescribe prevention. Insurance denies it. Patients can't afford it. Conditions worsen. Crises occur. Insurance pays for expensive treatment that could have been prevented for a fraction of the cost.

We know what works. We prescribe it. The system refuses to provide it. Then everyone acts surprised when preventable crises occur.

The frustration is profound. We're trained to prevent disease, keep people healthy, and intervene early. The system we work in is designed to wait for a crisis, then treat aggressively. We're constantly fighting against the system's incentives, trying to provide preventive care the system won't pay for, watching patients deteriorate because prevention was denied.

We're left watching insurance pay vastly more for treatment than they would have for prevention. The math is obvious. The evidence is clear, but profit doesn't come from prevention—it comes from treatment. So prevention gets denied, patients suffer, costs escalate, and the system profits from the very crises it could have prevented.

This is sick by design. Literally designed to keep people sick because sickness is profitable.

Why American Healthcare Stays Reactive

It's not ignorance. Everyone knows prevention works better. The evidence is overwhelming. Decades of research across multiple countries and healthcare systems prove that prevention costs less and achieves better outcomes. Healthcare executives, policy makers, physicians, economists—everyone involved in healthcare understands that prevention is superior to reaction.

We stay reactive anyway because reactive care is profitable and preventive care is not.

Changing to a preventive model would require:

Upfront investment with delayed returns. Prevention requires spending money now to avoid treatment costs years or decades later, but quarterly earnings reports measure this quarter's profits, not savings that materialize ten years from now. Insurance companies operate on short time horizons—patients switch insurers, investments in prevention benefit future insurers, not current ones.

A preventive model requires thinking in decades. The current system thinks in quarters. The financial incentives favor short-term profit over long-term savings.

Shifting power from specialists to primary care. Prevention happens in primary care. Specialists treat advanced disease. The U.S. healthcare system is specialist-dominated—specialists earn far more, have higher status, control more resources.

In 2017, specialist compensation averaged $399,300 compared to $247,300 for primary care physicians—a gap of $152,000. The payment structure rewards specialty procedures, not primary care prevention. Shifting to prevention would mean paying primary care doctors more and specialists less. Specialists control medical societies, hospital departments, and healthcare policy. They're not going to advocate for changes that reduce their income and status.

Reducing hospital admissions. Hospitals profit from filled beds. Every prevented hospitalization is lost revenue. Prevention reduces heart attacks, strokes, complications from chronic disease, and other conditions requiring hospitalization. This is good for patients—they stay healthier and avoid crisis. It's bad for hospitals—their revenue drops.

Hospitals lobby against policies that would reduce admissions. They oppose prevention programs that would keep people healthier. They fight payment models that reward health outcomes rather than treatment volume. Their business model depends on sick people needing hospitalization. Prevention threatens that model.

Reducing pharmaceutical use. Pharmaceutical companies profit from chronic disease requiring lifetime medication. Diabetes generates billions in insulin sales. Preventing diabetes eliminates those sales. Heart disease generates billions in cardiac medication sales. Preventing heart disease eliminates those sales.

Pharmaceutical companies have no financial interest in prevention that reduces medication use. They invest in developing new medications for existing diseases—not in preventing the diseases that require medication. Their business model requires sick people needing drugs. Prevention threatens that model.

Keeping people healthy. This is the fundamental contradiction: the American healthcare industry profits from sick people. Keeping people healthy reduces revenue across hospitals, pharmaceutical companies, specialists, medical device manufacturers, and every other entity that profits from treating illness.

A preventive model would keep people healthier, reduce disease burden, prevent complications, and result in substantially less need for healthcare services. This is ideal for patients and society—people are healthier and costs are lower. It's catastrophic for healthcare corporations—their revenue collapses.

Every major player in American healthcare loses money if the system shifts to prevention:

- Hospitals lose billions in revenue from prevented hospitalizations
- Pharmaceutical companies lose billions from preventing chronic disease
- Specialists lose billions from prevented acute interventions
- Medical device manufacturers lose billions from prevented procedures
- Insurance companies invest in prevention but don't capture the savings

The financial incentives are aligned against prevention across the entire industry. No powerful entity benefits from prevention. Every powerful entity benefits from reactive treatment of illness.

This is why the system stays reactive despite overwhelming evidence that prevention works better. It's not an accident. It's not ignorance. It's not inefficiency. It's the system responding rationally to its incentive structure.

We know prevention is better. We know it saves money. We know it improves outcomes. We're not doing it because the entities that would need to invest in prevention don't benefit from it. They benefit from expensive reactive treatment of preventable illness.

The system is designed to maximize revenue, not health. Prevention reduces revenue by keeping people healthy. Therefore, the system avoids prevention even though prevention would benefit patients and society.

This is sick by design—literally designed to profit from sickness rather than health. Changing it would require changing the fundamental financial incentives that make illness profitable. That would threaten trillions in revenue across the healthcare industry.

So the system stays reactive, Americans stay sicker than citizens of peer nations, costs remain nearly triple what other countries pay, and outcomes remain inferior. Not because we don't know better. Knowing better doesn't change the profit motive that drives every decision.

What Preventive Healthcare Would Require

Shifting from reactive to preventive healthcare isn't complicated. Other countries have done it successfully. The requirements are clear, documented, and proven effective. The United States knows exactly what would be required:

Universal coverage. Everyone must have healthcare access without financial barriers. If prevention is contingent on insurance coverage, employment status, or ability to pay, many people won't access it. Prevention works at the population level—you need everyone participating, not just people who can afford it.

Every developed nation with better outcomes than the U.S. has universal coverage. This isn't coincidence. Universal coverage is the foundation of preventive healthcare. You can't prevent disease in people who can't access care.

Free preventive services at point of care. No copays, no deductibles, no prior authorization, and no cost sharing for preventive care. Financial barriers prevent people from accessing preventive services even when they have insurance. A $50 copay for a preventive screening deters people on tight budgets. High deductibles mean people avoid care until deductibles are met.

Other countries provide comprehensive preventive services—screenings, vaccinations, health checks, risk assessments—at zero cost. Prevention is too important to leave contingent on whether people can afford copays.

Strong primary care infrastructure. Prevention happens in primary care through ongoing relationships between patients and primary care providers. The U.S. is specialist-dominant. Other countries with better outcomes are primary care-dominant.

This requires paying primary care physicians more, training more primary care doctors, supporting primary care practice infrastructure, and valuing generalist care as much as specialist interventions. It means reversing the payment structure that currently makes primary care the lowest-paid and lowest-status medical specialty.

Payment models that reward health outcomes, not treatment volume. As long as payment rewards procedures, hospital admissions, and treatment volume, the system will optimize for those activities. Paying for prevention requires changing how providers are compensated.

Other countries use capitation (payment per patient regardless of services provided), bundled payments (single payment for all care related to a condition), and outcome-based payments (bonuses for keeping populations healthy). These models incentivize prevention because providers profit from keeping patients healthy rather than treating illness.

Integration of medical, dental, vision, and mental health care. The U.S. fragments care by body system—medical insurance, dental insurance, vision insurance, and mental health carved out separately. This fragmentation prevents comprehensive prevention.

Dental disease causes heart problems. Vision problems cause falls. Mental health conditions manifest as physical illness. Treating the whole person rather than separating care by arbitrary body-system boundaries enables better prevention. Other countries integrate these services under universal coverage.

Community health workers for ongoing support. Chronic disease management, medication adherence, lifestyle support, early problem identification—these require ongoing engagement, not just episodic doctor visits. Community health workers provide this support in many universal healthcare systems.

They visit patients at home, help navigate healthcare systems, provide education and support, identify problems early, and keep people engaged with preventive care. This ongoing relationship enables prevention that isolated doctor appointments can't achieve.

Public health investment addressing social determinants. Healthcare alone doesn't determine health. Housing, food security, education, employment, environmental factors—these social determinants of health are often more important than medical care.

Countries with better outcomes invest in public health, address social determinants, and recognize that medical care operates within broader social context. The U.S. underfunds public health and ignores social determinants, then wonders why medical care alone doesn't keep people healthy.

System incentives aligned with health, not revenue. This is fundamental. As long as profit comes from treating illness, the system will optimize for illness. Aligning incentives with health means the system profits from keeping people healthy—through capitation, population health management, value-based care, or other models where provider success depends on patient health.

This requires removing profit extraction from healthcare or heavily regulating it. Other countries have non-profit universal systems or tightly regulate insurance companies and healthcare providers. The U.S. allows unrestricted profit extraction, creating incentives opposed to health.

These requirements are straightforward. They're not theoretical or untested. Every developed nation with better health outcomes than the U.S. has implemented them. They work. They're proven. They result in better health at lower cost.

The United States knows what's required. We're not doing it because implementing these changes would threaten healthcare industry profits. Insurance companies, hospitals, pharmaceutical companies, and specialists profit from the current reactive system. Prevention would reduce their revenue.

So we continue spending twice as much as peer nations while achieving worse outcomes. Not because we don't know what works. Because what works threatens profit, and profit is prioritized over health.

The Path Exists—We're Choosing Not to Take It

American healthcare doesn't lack solutions. We know what works. Every other developed nation demonstrates it daily. The path to better, cheaper healthcare is obvious, documented, and proven effective across dozens of countries and billions of people.

Universal coverage removes financial barriers to care. Emphasis on primary care and prevention keeps people healthy. Coordination of care prevents fragmentation. Payment models aligned with health outcomes incentivize prevention. Integration of medical, dental, vision, and mental health treats the whole person. Public health investment addresses social determinants.

Every peer nation does this. All achieve better outcomes spending half as much. The model exists. It works. It's not experimental or theoretical. It's the standard approach in the developed world—everywhere except the United States.

We know prevention works. Research proves it conclusively. Every dollar spent on prevention saves three to ten dollars in treatment costs. Preventing diabetes costs $500. Treating it costs $100,000+ over a lifetime. Preventing heart attacks costs $5,000. Treating them costs $150,000+. Preventing mental health crises costs $2,000. Treating them costs $50,000+.

The ROI is overwhelming. The evidence is undeniable. The path is clear.

We're not taking that path.

We're choosing reactive care that costs twice as much and achieves worse outcomes. We're choosing to let Americans die three years younger than citizens of peer nations. We're choosing infant mortality rates 60% higher than peer nations. We're choosing maternal mortality rates three to four times higher than peer nations. We're choosing chronic disease rates that dwarf other countries.

We're making these choices deliberately. Not because we don't know better, but because the current system is too profitable for too many powerful interests.

Insurance companies profit from the current system. They collect premiums, deny coverage, and extract billions in profit. Universal healthcare would eliminate their business model. They lobby aggressively against reform.

Pharmaceutical companies profit from the current system. They charge whatever they want for medications because the U.S. refuses to negotiate prices. Other countries negotiate nationally and pay half as much. Pharma companies fight any price controls.

Hospitals profit from the current system. They fill beds with preventable admissions, charge whatever insurance will pay, and generate massive revenue from treating illness. Prevention would reduce admissions and cut their income.

Specialists profit from the current system. They perform procedures on preventable conditions and earn far more than primary care physicians. Prevention would shift resources to primary care, reducing specialist income.

Every powerful entity in American healthcare opposes the changes that would improve outcomes and reduce costs. They profit from the current system. They lobby to preserve it. They fund politicians who oppose reform. They run advertising campaigns claiming universal healthcare would reduce quality or restrict choice.

The claims are lies. Every country with universal healthcare has better quality and more choice than Americans experience. These lies serve industry interests by preventing reform that would threaten profits.

The choice is stark: prevention or profit. Health or revenue. Better outcomes at lower cost, or worse outcomes at nearly triple the cost that generate maximum profit.

We're choosing profit. We've been choosing profit for decades. The result is Americans living shorter, sicker lives while paying twice as much as citizens of every peer nation.

This can change. The path exists. Other countries prove it works. We could implement universal healthcare that emphasizes prevention, costs half as much, and achieves better outcomes. We could do this within a few years if we chose to.

We're choosing not to. Not because it's impossible. Not because we don't know how, but because profit is prioritized over health, and the entities profiting from sickness have more political power than patients dying from preventable disease.

This is sick by design. The system is designed to maximize profit from treating illness rather than optimizing health through prevention. That design is killing Americans—literally killing us three years younger than we should live, killing babies at rates 60% higher than peer nations, killing mothers at rates three times higher than peer nations.

Every death from preventable disease, every medical bankruptcy, every person who couldn't access preventive care because they couldn't afford it—these are consequences of choosing profit over health.

The path to better healthcare exists. We're choosing not to take it. People are dying as a result. This is the choice America has made: let people die preventably rather than threaten healthcare industry profits.

We could choose differently. Every other developed nation has. We refuse because the current system, despite killing people and bankrupting families, is too profitable to change.

That's American healthcare: sick by design, profitable by intention, deadly by choice.

> *As I've argued so far, this is a choice. We can still find our way out of this trap and onto the path towards better health. That starts with a clear vision of what could be. As a nation built by dreamers, that is something we should be more than capable of.*

Research Notes:

This chapter synthesizes international healthcare comparisons from peer-reviewed literature documenting U.S. spending at nearly double peer nations ($14,775 vs. $7,860 per capita mean in 2024), worse outcomes across life expectancy (78.8 years vs. 81.7 mean), infant mortality (5.8 per 1,000 vs. 3.6 mean), and maternal mortality (highest in developed world). Healthcare spending grew 7.5% in 2023—the highest rate since 2003 outside the pandemic, outpacing GDP growth. ROI data on preventive interventions demonstrates $3-10 saved per dollar invested. The fundamental finding: higher U.S. spending reflects pricing failure rather than utilization differences, with administrative costs at 8% vs. 1-3% in other nations and pharmaceutical spending at $1,443 per capita vs. $466-939 in peer countries. Personal perspectives integrate clinical experience with denied preventive care and connections between inadequate mental health access and societal crises.

CHAPTER 12

Breaking Free

What Healthcare Could Be

The following scenario describes how healthcare works in every developed nation except the United States. For Americans, it reads like science fiction. For everyone else, it's Tuesday.

Sarah Chen felt the lump in her breast on a Monday morning. By Monday afternoon, she'd seen her primary care doctor. By Tuesday, she'd had a mammogram and ultrasound. By Wednesday, a biopsy confirmed breast cancer. By the following Monday—eight days after finding the lump—she'd met with an oncologist, reviewed her treatment options, and scheduled surgery for the following week.

She didn't call her insurance company. She didn't check if the oncologist was in-network. She didn't calculate whether she'd met her deductible. She didn't start a GoFundMe campaign. She didn't worry about losing her job and her coverage. She didn't delay treatment while fighting claim denials or waiting for prior authorization.

She focused on one thing: getting healthy.

The surgery went well. Chemotherapy followed.

Six months of treatment, dozens of appointments, multiple specialists, extensive imaging, laboratory work, medications. She received excellent care from providers who spent their time on medicine rather than billing codes and insurance paperwork.

When it was over, Sarah had beaten cancer. She had her health, her job, her home, and her savings. She hadn't received a single medical bill. Not one. The only financial impact was missing some work during treatment—and her job was protected by law, with income replacement ensuring her family didn't face financial crisis while she healed.

This isn't fantasy. This isn't utopian imagination. This is exactly how cancer treatment works in Canada, the UK, France, Germany, Japan, Australia, and every other developed nation except the United States.

Americans can't imagine this experience because we've never had it. We can't conceive of healthcare without the constant background terror of financial catastrophe. We can't picture medical care where the only question is "What treatment do you need?" rather than "How will you pay for it?"

This is normal everywhere else. It's how healthcare works when systems are designed to promote health rather than generate profit. It's what happens when coverage is universal, costs are controlled, and the goal is keeping people healthy rather than extracting maximum revenue from illness.

Sarah Chen's story could be any American's story—if we chose to build a healthcare system that served patients rather than shareholders. The system exists. It works. Dozens of countries prove it daily.

We just have to choose it.

Universal Healthcare: The Actual Definition

Americans hear "universal healthcare" and imagine government bureaucrats deciding who gets care, long wait times, poor quality, and loss of choice. This is industry propaganda, not reality. Let's define what universal healthcare actually means.

Universal healthcare means everyone is covered. Every resident has access to comprehensive medical care without financial barriers. Coverage isn't contingent on employment, income, health status, or ability to pay. You're covered because you exist, because you're a resident or a citizen, because healthcare is treated as a right rather than a commodity.

Universal healthcare does NOT mean the government running everything. Multiple models achieve universal coverage. Some have government-provided care (like the UK's NHS). Others use private insurance heavily regulated to ensure universal access (like Germany or Switzerland). Others mix public coverage with private options (like Australia). The specific structure varies. The principle doesn't: everyone gets healthcare.

Universal healthcare is financed through taxes, not premiums and deductibles. Instead of paying insurance companies, you pay taxes. The difference is progressive taxation means wealthy people pay more, while current insurance premiums are regressive—everyone pays similar amounts regardless of income. A family earning $40,000 and a family earning $400,000 might both pay $15,000 annually for insurance. Under universal healthcare, the wealthy family pays far more, the middle-class family pays less, and the poor family pays little or nothing.

Universal healthcare regulates prices. Governments negotiate with providers, hospitals, and pharmaceutical companies. They set reimbursement rates. They control costs. This is why other countries spend half as much per capita—not because they provide less care but because they don't allow unlimited profit extraction from healthcare.

Universal healthcare focuses on health outcomes, not revenue. Success is measured by population health—life expectancy, infant mortality, disease rates, quality of life. Not by hospital occupancy rates, procedure volumes, or profit margins. When the system's goal is health, prevention becomes priority. When the goal is revenue, treatment of illness becomes priority.

That's universal healthcare: everyone covered, financed through progressive taxation, prices regulated to prevent profit extraction, focused on health rather than revenue. The specifics vary by country. The principles don't.

This works. Every developed nation except the United States has proven this for decades. Better outcomes, lower costs, no medical bankruptcy, nobody avoiding care because they can't afford it. Not theory. Reality.

Single-Payer Model: Medicare for All

Single-payer healthcare means one government insurance program covering everyone. The government collects taxes, pays for care, and negotiates prices with providers. Everyone gets the same comprehensive coverage. No premiums, no deductibles, no copays—or minimal cost-sharing that doesn't create access barriers.

Canada's provincial single-payer system demonstrates how this works. Thirteen provincial and territorial governments operate tax-funded public insurance plans providing universal coverage for medically necessary physician and hospital services, free at point of care. It's not technically a national system—it's provincial systems meeting national standards, but coverage is portable across the entire country.

Canadians choose any doctor, any hospital. No networks. No prior authorization for most care. No fighting insurance companies over coverage. You show your provincial health card and receive care. Hospitals are funded by provincial governments. Physicians submit claims and get paid promptly with almost no preapproval or administrative barriers.

The system is characterized by extraordinarily low administrative costs and simple enrollment. Virtually everyone with legal status in Canada easily acquires a card with neither complex enrollment nor extensive paperwork. Hospitals collect funds from the government with low reporting costs. Physicians are paid with minimal bureaucracy—the opposite of American providers spending hours on insurance paperwork.

Canada achieves this with government health spending of 7.4% of GDP—less than the OECD mean of 8.3%. The vast majority of Canadians have access to primary care with continuity. Cancer survival rates are among the world's highest. Patients don't go bankrupt from medical bills—it doesn't happen in Canada. Healthcare costs are a non-issue for Canadian families.

What should be said, is that Canada does have wait times for elective care. In 2016, 30% of Canadians waited more than two months for specialist referrals—higher than any OECD comparator.

Similarly, 18% waited more than four months for elective non-urgent surgery. If you need hip replacement, cataract surgery, or other elective procedures, you might wait months.

However—and this is critical—urgent medical and surgical care is timely. Heart attacks, strokes, cancer, emergencies: immediate treatment. The wait times apply to elective procedures that aren't urgent. Importantly, these wait times don't translate to worse health outcomes. Canada ranked 17th globally on the Healthcare Access and Quality Index based on mortality from amenable causes, compared to the UK at 30th and the US at 35th.

Americans need to understand: Canada's wait times exist for non-urgent elective procedures. Urgent care is immediate. Canada achieves better health outcomes at half the cost despite those wait times. Meanwhile, Americans face our own wait times—financial waits. We delay care we can't afford, often until conditions become severe enough to require emergency treatment. That delay causes worse outcomes than Canada's scheduling waits.

The United Kingdom's National Health Service goes beyond single-payer insurance to government provision of care. The NHS doesn't just pay for healthcare—it owns hospitals and employs many doctors. Care is completely free at the point of service. No bills. No charges. Even visitors receive emergency care free.

The UK spent $3,825 per capita on healthcare in 2017—the least among comparable countries, less than half U.S. spending. The NHS is funded through general taxation. Everyone is covered automatically as a UK resident.

The NHS achieves the lowest rates of unmet healthcare need among comparator countries, despite having among the lowest numbers of doctors and nurses per capita. Outcomes are mixed—life expectancy slightly below average, cancer survival below average, but some excellent service outcomes like low healthcare-associated infections and reduced postoperative complications.

The NHS demonstrates that comprehensive universal coverage costs far less than the U.S. system, but it also shows that underfunding creates problems. Conservative governments have deliberately underfunded the NHS to make it appear dysfunctional, setting up arguments for privatization. When properly funded, the NHS delivers excellent care at minimal cost. When starved of resources, it struggles—but still outperforms the U.S. system on most metrics.

Single-payer advantages are substantial:

- Simplest administratively: one insurer, one set of rules, minimal bureaucracy
- Most equitable: everyone gets same coverage regardless of income or employment
- Lowest cost: administrative expenses of 1-3% versus 15-20% for private insurance
- Government leverage: can negotiate drug prices, set provider rates, control costs
- No medical bankruptcy: literally cannot happen under single-payer
- Free choice of provider: no networks restricting which doctors you can see

Single-payer disadvantages are mostly political, not practical:

- Threatens insurance industry existence—generates massive lobbying opposition
- Requires overcoming propaganda about "government takeover"
- May have wait times for elective procedures (though urgent care remains immediate)
- Politically difficult in U.S. despite working successfully in multiple countries

The evidence is clear: single-payer works. Canada, UK, Taiwan, and other countries prove it delivers better outcomes at lower cost. Americans fear it because industry propaganda has convinced us that government insurance means poor quality and restricted access. The reality is opposite: single-payer provides better access and comparable or better quality at half the cost.

Medicare—the existing U.S. government insurance for people 65 and older—has 2% overhead versus 15-20% for private insurance. Beneficiaries consistently rate Medicare highly. The infrastructure exists. We could expand it to cover everyone. The only obstacle is political will and industry opposition.

Multi-Payer Universal Model: Regulated Private Insurance

Single-payer isn't the only path to universal healthcare. Multiple countries achieve universal coverage through heavily regulated private insurance. Everyone must have insurance, but multiple insurance companies compete under strict rules ensuring comprehensive, affordable coverage for all residents.

Germany's system provides the clearest example. Approximately 90% of Germans are covered by statutory health insurance (SHI) through nonprofit "sickness funds"—quasi-public insurance entities heavily regulated by the government. The remaining 10%, mostly high earners, opt for private insurance.

Everyone must have coverage—the individual mandate is actually enforced. Premiums are income-based, approximately 15% of income split between employers and employees. This progressive financing means wealthy people pay more, poor people pay less—the opposite of U.S. insurance where everyone pays similar premiums regardless of income.

Coverage is comprehensive. No pre-existing condition exclusions, no lifetime caps, no coverage denials for medical necessity. Minimal cost-sharing that doesn't create access barriers. Germans have free choice of sickness fund and free choice of providers. Strong primary care, excellent outcomes, moderate costs.

Wait times in Germany are minimal. Only 3% of Germans waited more than two months to see a specialist—compared to 39% in Canada or 19% in the UK. The regulated multi-payer system delivers timely access that rivals or exceeds single-payer systems.

France's system works similarly. Universal statutory health insurance supplemented by voluntary complementary insurance that approximately 95% of people have. Government sets coverage requirements and reimbursement rates. Very low out-of-pocket costs. Consistently ranks among the world's best healthcare systems.

Wait times in France: 4% waited more than two months for specialist access. Essentially immediate care for most people while maintaining universal coverage.

Switzerland and the Netherlands use similar approaches—mandatory insurance, heavy regulation, subsidies ensuring affordability, comprehensive coverage requirements, no denials. Wait times: Switzerland 9%, Netherlands 7% waiting more than two months for specialists.

The pattern is clear: heavily regulated multi-payer systems can achieve universal coverage with excellent access and short wait times. They're more complex administratively than single-payer but preserve competition among insurers while ensuring everyone is covered.

Multi-payer advantages:

- Preserves insurance industry (reduces political opposition)
- Allows patient choice among competing insurers
- Can achieve very short wait times (Germany, France, Netherlands outperform single-payer on this metric)
- Demonstrates that universal coverage doesn't require eliminating private insurance

Multi-payer disadvantages:

- More administratively complex than single-payer
- Requires strong, sustained government regulation

- Higher administrative costs than single-payer (though still far less than U.S.)
- Potential for insurers to game regulations if enforcement is weak

The critical lesson: it's not single-payer versus multi-payer that matters. It's universal coverage with strong price regulation versus our current system of profit-driven insurance with minimal regulation. Germany, France, Switzerland, and the Netherlands prove that heavily regulated private insurance can deliver universal coverage with excellent outcomes—if the government enforces rules preventing profit extraction at the expense of coverage.

Hybrid Models: Mix of Public and Private

Some countries combine universal public coverage with optional private insurance, creating hybrid systems that guarantee everyone has comprehensive care while preserving private options for those who want them.

Australia's Medicare provides the clearest example. Australia has universal public insurance covering all residents—the actual Medicare that America named our program after. Everyone has comprehensive coverage automatically. Free hospital care, subsidized physician visits, prescription drug coverage through the Pharmaceutical Benefits Scheme.

Additionally, Australians can purchase private insurance for faster access to elective surgery, private hospital rooms, and services not fully covered by public Medicare. About half of Australians have private insurance. Higher earners face a surcharge if they don't maintain private coverage, creating incentive for the wealthy to buy private insurance rather than solely using the public system.

The key: the public system is robust enough that private insurance is truly optional. You're not forced into private coverage to get adequate care. Public Medicare provides comprehensive coverage. Private insurance offers choice and faster access to elective procedures—but nobody goes without care because they can't afford private coverage.

Australia achieves this spending approximately $5,000 per capita—a little over a half of U.S. spending. Life expectancy exceeds the U.S. by three years. Infant mortality is substantially lower. No medical bankruptcy. Better outcomes at half the cost, with universal public coverage as foundation and private insurance as optional enhancement.

Hybrid advantages:

- Universal public coverage ensures nobody goes without care
- Optional private insurance preserves choice for those who want it
- Political compromise: universal base satisfies progressives, private option satisfies moderates/ conservatives
- Prevents two-tier system if public coverage is adequately funded

Hybrid disadvantages:

- Risk of creating two-tier system if public coverage is underfunded

- More complex than pure single-payer
- Requires maintaining both public and private systems
- Private insurance may cream-skim healthiest patients, leaving sicker patients in public system

The hybrid model demonstrates that universal coverage and private insurance aren't mutually exclusive. You can have a robust public system ensuring everyone has care while allowing private insurance for additional services or faster access. The critical requirement: adequate public funding so the universal base provides genuine comprehensive coverage, not bare-minimum care that forces people into private insurance to get adequate treatment.

What These Systems Have in Common

Despite structural differences—single-payer, multi-payer, hybrid—all successful universal healthcare systems share fundamental characteristics:

Everyone is covered. No exclusions for pre-existing conditions. No denials based on health status. No uninsured population. Coverage is universal, comprehensive, and continuous. You're covered because you're a resident, not because you're employed or wealthy.

Coverage based on residency, not employment. Healthcare isn't tied to jobs. You don't lose coverage when you change employment, start a business, or retire before 65. This seems obvious in other countries—why would healthcare depend on who you work for? Only in America is employer-based coverage normal. Everywhere else recognized that tying healthcare to employment is irrational and harmful.

Minimal or no financial barriers at point of care. Some countries have small copays. Most don't. The principle: cost shouldn't prevent accessing necessary care. Compare this to American deductibles of $6,000-8,000 before insurance pays anything. Financial barriers in universal systems are negligible or nonexistent.

Government regulation of prices. All universal systems regulate what providers, hospitals, and pharmaceutical companies can charge. They negotiate prices. They set reimbursement rates. They prevent unlimited profit extraction. This is why they spend half as much as the U.S.—not because they provide less care but because they don't allow healthcare to be an unregulated marketplace where corporations charge whatever they want.

Emphasis on primary care and prevention. Universal systems invest in keeping people healthy because the system bears costs of illness. Prevention saves money when you're paying for treatment later. The U.S. does the opposite: prevention costs insurers money that different insurers might save later. Universal systems align incentives with health.

Non-profit or heavily regulated insurance. Whether single-payer government insurance, heavily regulated private insurance, or hybrid systems, profit extraction is eliminated or minimized. Insurance exists to pay for care, not generate corporate profits. This is fundamental: when insurance is non-profit or tightly regulated, administrative costs drop and coverage improves.

Progressive financing. Universal systems are funded through progressive taxation or income-based premiums. Wealthy people pay more, poor people pay less. U.S. insurance premiums are regressive—everyone pays similar amounts regardless of income. Universal systems finance healthcare equitably.

No medical bankruptcy. This doesn't exist in universal healthcare systems. Medical debt doesn't bankrupt families in Canada, UK, France, Germany, Japan, or anywhere else with universal coverage. It's uniquely American—the only developed nation where getting sick can destroy you financially even when you have insurance.

Lower administrative costs. Administrative expenses in universal systems range from 1-3% for single-payer to slightly higher for multi-payer, but all dramatically lower than the 15-20% overhead of U.S. private insurance or the 34.2% total administrative costs when including provider billing costs. Less bureaucracy, less paperwork, and more money for actual care.

Better health outcomes. Countries with universal healthcare have longer life expectancy, lower infant mortality, lower maternal mortality, better management of chronic disease, and better overall population health than the United States. This is consistent across all universal systems regardless of structure.

Lower costs. Every country with universal healthcare spends substantially less per capita than the United States. Peer countries average $7,860 versus our $14,775. Universal healthcare costs about half as much while covering everyone and achieving better outcomes.

The model details matter less than these shared principles. Single-payer, multi-payer, hybrid—all work when they ensure universal coverage, regulate prices, remove financial barriers, and focus on health rather than profit.

The lesson for America: we don't need to perfectly replicate any specific country's system. We need to implement these core principles:

- Cover everyone
- Regulate prices
- Remove financial barriers
- Focus on health

Any model incorporating these principles will work better and cost less than our current profit-driven system.

Addressing Common Objections: "But Wait Times!"

The most common objection to universal healthcare: "You'll have to wait months for care! Rationing! Government bureaucrats deciding when you can see doctors!"

Let's examine reality rather than propaganda.

Wait times exist in U.S. healthcare. Average wait for primary care appointments in the U.S.: 31 days in 2025. That's four weeks to see your primary care doctor for routine appointments. Americans already wait. We just don't call it rationing when the wait is caused by provider shortages rather than system design.

International wait time comparison for specialists: The percentage of people waiting more than two months to see a specialist:

- United States: 6%
- Germany: 3%

- France: 4%
- Netherlands: 7%
- Switzerland: 9%
- UK: 19%
- Canada: 39%

The U.S. performs well—better than the UK and Canada, similar to insurance-based European systems. That said, we're not dramatically better than heavily regulated multi-payer systems in Germany, France, and the Netherlands.

Emergency care is immediate everywhere. Heart attacks, strokes, serious injuries, cancer, urgent medical needs—these are treated immediately in all developed countries including those with universal coverage. The wait times people reference apply to elective procedures that aren't urgent. Hip replacement, cataract surgery, non-urgent diagnostic imaging—these might have waits in some universal systems.

Americans have financial wait times instead. We don't schedule appointments we can't afford. We delay care because we haven't met deductibles. We put off seeing doctors until symptoms become unbearable. These are wait times—just financial rather than scheduling.

Before the pandemic, 44% of Americans delayed care due to cost. That's a wait time. That's rationing. That's being unable to access healthcare you need. It just happens through price rather than scheduling, so we don't call it rationing.

And financial wait times cause worse outcomes than scheduling waits. Delaying cancer screening because you can't afford the copay means cancer progresses to later stages requiring more aggressive treatment. Delaying cardiac care because you haven't met your deductible means heart attacks that could have been prevented. Financial waits kill people. Scheduling waits for elective procedures are inconvenient but don't generally cause worse health outcomes.

Why do Canada and the UK have longer waits than European multi-payer systems? Provider supply. Canada and the UK have fewer doctors per capita than insurance-based European systems. The wait times reflect provider shortages, not inherent flaws in single-payer or national health service models.

Importantly, Canada's wait times don't translate to worse outcomes. Canada ranks 17th globally on Healthcare Access and Quality Index based on mortality from amenable causes—substantially better than the U.S. at 35th. The waits exist but don't prevent Canada from achieving better health outcomes than America.

If the U.S. implemented universal healthcare, would wait times increase? Probably not for most care. We'd likely see:

- Improved access to primary care as more people could afford routine visits
- Reduced emergency room overcrowding as people access primary care instead of using ER for routine problems
- More people seeking preventive care (currently delayed due to cost)
- Potential need to expand provider workforce to

accommodate newly insured population

The American Medical Association and other provider organizations have opposed universal coverage partly because increased access would mean more work, but that's a feature, not a bug. People are currently going without needed care. Universal coverage would let them access that care. We'd need to train more providers—which universal systems can afford because they save hundreds of billions on administration.

The wait time objection is propaganda. It ignores that Americans already wait. It ignores financial barriers that prevent accessing care entirely. It ignores that universal systems achieve better health outcomes despite occasional waits for elective procedures. It presents scheduling waits as intolerable while ignoring the financial waits that kill people.

Emergency care is immediate in universal systems. Urgent care is prioritized. Elective procedures might have waits in some systems, particularly those that underfund their public coverage. But nobody goes without necessary care because they can't afford it. Nobody delays cancer screening until too late because of deductibles. Nobody dies from preventable conditions because insurance denied coverage.

Trade a few weeks' wait for elective hip replacement for immediate access to all necessary care with no financial barriers? Most Americans would make that trade happily—if they understood that's the actual choice, not the propaganda version claiming universal healthcare means dying while waiting for government permission to see doctors.

Addressing Common Objections: "Government Bureaucracy!"

"Universal healthcare means government bureaucracy! DMV-level inefficiency! Endless paperwork! Government between you and your doctor!"

This objection would be laughable if it weren't so widely believed. The U.S. healthcare system is the most bureaucratic, administratively complex, paperwork-intensive system in the developed world. What Americans imagine universal healthcare might be like is exactly what we currently have.

Administrative costs in U.S. versus universal systems:

- U.S. administrative costs (narrow definition): 8% of healthcare spending
- U.S. administrative costs (comprehensive): 34.2% of healthcare spending—$812 billion annually, $2,497 per capita
- Canada administrative costs: 17.0% of spending—$551 per capita
- Single-payer systems: 1-3% overhead

Let that sink in. American healthcare spends 34.2% of every healthcare dollar on administration. Canada spends 17.0%. Single-payer government insurance typically spends 1-3%. The most bureaucratic healthcare systems in the world are private insurance-based systems like ours. Government-run insurance is dramatically more efficient.

Medicare versus private insurance overhead:

- Medicare Parts A, B, and D: 1.35% administrative expenses
- Medicare Advantage (private insurance): 10.86-14.84% administrative expenses
- Private insurance generally: 15-20% overhead

U.S. government insurance (Medicare) is 8-11 times more efficient than private insurance. The bureaucracy Americans fear from government-run healthcare is a fraction of the bureaucracy we currently endure from private insurance.

What creates U.S. healthcare bureaucracy?

Prior authorization requirements. Claim denials and appeals. Billing disputes. Checking whether providers are in-network. Understanding deductibles, coinsurance, out-of-pocket maximums. Medical coding for billing. Fighting insurance companies over coverage. Calling to verify benefits. Submitting claims. Following up on unpaid claims. Appealing denials. Documentation for prior authorization. Peer-to-peer reviews. Utilization review.

This is what American healthcare providers spend one-third of their time doing: administrative tasks related to insurance. Not patient care. Insurance paperwork.

- Billing costs per encounter in the U.S.:

- Primary care visit: $20.49
- Emergency department visit: $61.54
- npatient hospital stay: $124.26
- Outpatient surgical procedure: $170.40
- Inpatient surgical procedure: $215.10

Every single medical encounter in America generates massive administrative costs just for billing and insurance. In Canada, billing costs per inpatient surgical encounter: $6. In the U.S.: $215. That's not a typo—American billing costs are 36 times higher.

The bureaucracy isn't the government. It's private insurance creating complex, fragmented, claim-denying systems that require armies of administrators to navigate.

Universal healthcare has LESS bureaucracy:

Single set of rules, not hundreds of different insurance policies

No prior authorization for most care—doctor says you need it, you get it

- No claim denials to fight—everything medically necessary is covered
- No network restrictions—see any provider
- No checking if services are covered—they are
- No billing disputes—providers are paid according to standard fee schedules

- No need for patients to understand complex insurance terms

Providers in universal systems spend their time on medicine. They're not fighting insurance companies. They're not documenting justifications for prior authorization. They're not coding for optimal billing. They're treating patients.

"Keep the government out of my Medicare" isn't just a joke. It's revealing. Americans love Medicare. Beneficiaries consistently rate it highly. Medicare has less bureaucracy, better coverage, and lower administrative costs than private insurance. When Americans say they don't want government healthcare, they're revealing they don't understand that Medicare—which they love—is government healthcare.

The real bureaucracy problem: profit-driven insurance companies denying claims to maximize revenue. Government insurance doesn't deny claims for profit—it covers what's medically necessary. That's less bureaucratic, not more.

Electronic health records: Americans were told EHRs would reduce paperwork. They haven't. Administrative costs continue rising. Why? Because EHRs were implemented in a fragmented private insurance system requiring extensive documentation for billing and denial prevention. In universal systems, EHRs can actually reduce administration because there's no need to document defensively against insurance denials.

The bureaucracy objection is projection. Americans fear universal healthcare will be bureaucratic like our current system. Yet, the reason our current system is bureaucratic is because it's profit-driven private insurance. Government-run insurance is demonstrably less bureaucratic, more efficient, and easier to navigate.

Ask any American who's eligible for Medicare: would you trade Medicare for private insurance? Almost none would. Medicare is government bureaucracy, and it's vastly superior to private insurance bureaucracy.

Addressing Common Objections: "Loss of Choice!"

"Universal healthcare restricts your choice of doctors! The government decides what treatments you can have! You can't choose your insurance!"

This objection is backwards. Americans have dramatically less choice than citizens of universal healthcare countries.

Choice of doctors

United States: You can only see doctors in your insurance network. Out-of-network care costs dramatically more or isn't covered at all. Change jobs, change insurance, lose access to your doctors. Can't afford insurance, can't see any doctors.

Canada: Choose any doctor, any hospital, anywhere in the country. No network restrictions. No referral requirements for most care. True free choice of providers.

Germany, France, UK, most universal systems: Free choice of providers. No network restrictions in most countries. Your ability to see a doctor isn't determined by which insurance company you have.

Americans think we have a choice because we can theoretically choose between insurance plans—if we can afford them, if our employer offers them, or if we can understand the differences. In reality, that's not healthcare choice. That's choosing which restrictions to accept.

In universal systems, you choose doctors. Not insurance plans. Not networks. Doctors.

Choice of treatments

United States: Insurance companies decide what treatments they'll cover. Prior authorization required for many treatments. Claim denials common. Experimental or expensive treatments often denied. Medications restricted by insurance formularies. Treatments decided by insurance company employees who've never examined you, often overruling your doctor's recommendations.

Universal systems: Treatments decided by doctors and patients. No insurance company approval needed for medically necessary care. Evidence-based guidelines exist (just like in the U.S.), but doctors have more autonomy. No profit motive driving denials.

Who would you rather make treatment decisions: your doctor, or an insurance company employee whose bonus depends on denying expensive treatments?

Choice of insurance

United States: You get what your employer offers. Can't afford employer insurance or don't have employer coverage? Buy marketplace insurance if you can afford it. Don't like your insurance? Too bad—you can't switch outside enrollment periods, can't afford better plans, so you're stuck with what you have.

Universal systems: Everyone has coverage automatically. In multi-payer systems like Germany, you can choose among competing insurers—but all are required to provide comprehensive coverage, so the differences are minimal. In single-payer systems, everyone has the same coverage—which means nobody has better coverage than you because they're wealthier.

Real choice is about accessing care, not selecting among inadequate insurance options. Universal systems provide choice where it matters: choosing doctors and receiving treatments. American insurance restricts both while pretending that choosing among bad insurance options constitutes a meaningful choice.

Treatment restrictions

U.S. insurance companies deny treatments constantly:

- "Not medically necessary" (despite doctor saying it is)
- "Experimental" (even for FDA-approved treatments)
- "Not covered under your plan"
- Prior authorization delays or denials
- Step therapy requirements (try cheaper options first even when doctor says you need specific treatment)

Universal systems have treatment guidelines based on clinical evidence, but doctors can deviate when medically justified. There's no profit motive driving denial. If treatment is medically necessary and evidence-based, it's provided.

The freedom to choose suffering:

America offers one choice universal systems don't: the choice to go without healthcare because you can't afford it. You can choose to avoid necessary care because of deductibles, skip medications because they're too expensive, or go bankrupt from medical bills.

These aren't choices. They're failures of the healthcare system masquerading as freedom.

Real healthcare choice means choosing doctors, accessing treatments, making medical decisions with your physicians. Universal systems provide these choices. The American system restricts them while claiming that insurance company networks and formularies constitute choice.

Americans who've experienced both systems:

People who've lived in the U.S. and countries with universal healthcare consistently report having *more* choice in universal systems. They could see any doctor without checking networks. They didn't fight for coverage. They made medical decisions without insurance company interference.

Americans living abroad often cite healthcare as a reason they don't want to return to the U.S. They've experienced actual healthcare choice—and they don't want to trade it for American insurance restrictions.

The choice objection is propaganda. It claims universal healthcare restricts choice while ignoring that American insurance restricts choice far more. It pretends selecting among inadequate insurance options is freedom while universal systems provide the only choice that matters: access to care when you need it.

Addressing Common Objections: "It's Too Expensive!"

"We can't afford universal healthcare! It would cost trillions! Taxes would skyrocket! It's economically impossible!"

This objection reveals complete ignorance of healthcare economics. We can't afford NOT to have universal healthcare. The current system costs twice as much as universal systems while covering fewer people and achieving worse outcomes.

The spending comparison:

- U.S. spending per capita: $14,775
- Countries with universal healthcare: $6,747 to $9,963
- U.S. spending as percent of GDP: 17.8%
- Universal healthcare countries: 9.6-12.4%

We're already paying more than enough for universal healthcare. We spend almost double what countries with universal coverage spend. If we implemented universal healthcare and matched other countries' costs, we'd save trillions while covering everyone.

Medicare for All cost studies:

A systematic review of 22 economic analyses of single-payer plans found that 19 (86%) predicted net savings in the first year and 20 (91%) predicted savings over several years. Median savings: 3.46% of total healthcare costs.

A 2020 Lancet study calculated Medicare for All would lead to 13% savings in national healthcare expenditure—equivalent to more than $450 billion annually. The entire system could be funded with less money than current spending by employers and households on premiums combined with existing government allocations.

Another analysis estimated $375 billion in annual administrative savings alone—nearly 15% of healthcare spending—from simplified financing compared to our current multi-payer system.

Even the "Koch brothers study"—funded by libertarian opponents of universal healthcare to prove it would be expensive—concluded it would save money. Industry-funded research designed to show universal healthcare was unaffordable ended up proving it would reduce costs. The evidence is overwhelming: universal healthcare costs less than our current system.

Where the savings come from:

Administrative efficiency: Eliminate $375-471 billion in billing and insurance-related costs. Single-payer overhead of 1-3% versus private insurance overhead of 15-20%. Massive reduction in provider administrative burden.

Drug price negotiation: Save $100+ billion annually by negotiating pharmaceutical prices like every other country does. We're currently prohibited from negotiating Medicare drug prices. Eliminating that prohibition and negotiating nationally would save enormous amounts.

Reduced profit extraction: Eliminate insurance company profits. Eliminate pharmaceutical company excess profits from price gouging. Eliminate hospital corporate profits from overcharging. The money currently extracted as profit can pay for expanding coverage.

Prevention emphasis: Keep people healthier, reduce expensive acute care, prevent complications from chronic disease. Universal systems invest in prevention because they capture the savings. We don't because patients switch insurers before savings materialize.

How to pay for it:

Replace premiums, deductibles, copays, and out-of-pocket spending with progressive taxation. Most people would pay less under universal healthcare than they currently pay for insurance.

Example calculation: Family currently paying $15,000 annually in premiums plus $6,000 deductible = $21,000 total healthcare spending. Under Medicare for All with progressive income tax of 4% on income over $29,000:

- Family earning $60,000 pays approximately $1,240 in healthcare tax
- Saves $19,760 annually compared to current spending

Only the wealthy would pay more—which is appropriate since they can afford it. Working and middle-class families would save money. The poor would pay little or nothing.

"How do we pay for it?" is propaganda:

We're already paying for it. Twice over. We're spending $14,775 per capita on healthcare—more than enough to fund universal coverage if costs were controlled like other countries control costs. Healthcare spending grew 7.5% in 2023 alone, outpacing economic growth, proving the current system is financially unsustainable.

The question isn't "How do we pay for universal healthcare?" It's "Why are we paying twice as much for worse outcomes?" Or perhaps more importantly "Can we afford to continue the current system that's bankrupting families and killing people?"

Employer savings:

Employers currently spending thousands per employee on insurance would save money under Medicare for All. No more insurance premiums. No more administrative costs of managing benefits. They'd pay payroll taxes instead—likely lower than current insurance costs.

Small businesses would benefit enormously. They struggle to afford insurance for employees. Universal healthcare eliminates that cost, making them more competitive with large corporations.

Economic impact:

Healthcare destabilization and costs are harming the U.S. economy. Medical bankruptcy affects 530,000 families annually. People trapped in jobs they hate because of insurance. Entrepreneurship suppressed. People avoiding care until conditions become severe and expensive.

Universal healthcare would free people from job lock, enable entrepreneurship, eliminate medical bankruptcy, reduce economic anxiety, and make American businesses more competitive globally by eliminating employer healthcare costs.

The "too expensive" objection is absurd. We're already spending far more than universal healthcare would cost. We'd save hundreds of billions annually while covering everyone and achieving better outcomes.

The real question isn't cost. It's whether we're willing to challenge insurance company profits, pharmaceutical company profits, and hospital corporate profits to implement a system that serves people instead of shareholders.

We can afford universal healthcare. We can't afford to continue without it.

Addressing Common Objections: "Quality Will Suffer!"

"Universal healthcare means lower quality care! America has the best healthcare in the world! Other countries ration care and have worse outcomes!"

This objection requires examining what "quality" means and what outcomes actually show.

Health outcomes in U.S. versus universal healthcare countries:

- Life expectancy: U.S. 78.8 years, universal healthcare countries 80.7-83.9 years (mean 81.7)
- Infant mortality: U.S. 5.8 per 1,000 live births, universal healthcare countries 1.8-4.0 (mean 3.6)
- Maternal mortality: U.S. 32.9 per 100,000 live births, most universal healthcare countries under 10
- Chronic disease rates: U.S. has higher rates of diabetes, heart disease, obesity than peer nations

Americans die younger. Our babies die more frequently. Our mothers die at three to four times the rate of peer nations. We have worse outcomes across nearly every measure.

This isn't “the best healthcare in the world." This is substantially worse healthcare than every other developed nation.

That said, American acute care IS excellent:

The U.S. excels at treating medical emergencies for people who can access care. Trauma care, emergency cardiac interventions, cancer treatment for advanced disease—American medicine is world-class.

The problem: we're excellent at treating illness but terrible at preventing it. We wait for people to get sick, then deploy extraordinary interventions. Other countries prevent illness, catch disease early, manage chronic conditions effectively—and as a result need less acute care.

Our acute care excellence doesn't compensate for our prevention failure. Better to prevent heart attacks than treat them brilliantly. Better to catch cancer early than treat advanced disease with cutting-edge therapies. Better to manage diabetes to prevent complications than treat complications after they develop.

Quality metrics favor universal systems:

When you measure what matters—life expectancy, infant mortality, maternal mortality, disease burden, quality of life—universal systems outperform the U.S. consistently. We can't claim quality superiority when Americans are dying younger and babies are dying more frequently.

Even privileged Americans have worse health:

White Americans in the highest-income counties—the most advantaged population in the United States—have worse health outcomes than average residents of other developed countries. The U.S. health disadvantage isn't explained by poverty or poor health behaviors among disadvantaged populations. Even our healthiest, wealthiest citizens have worse outcomes than middle-class citizens of peer nations.

Medical innovation:

Industry argues that universal healthcare would reduce medical innovation. In reality, the most basic research is government-funded through NIH and similar agencies. Pharmaceutical companies develop drugs, but often based on publicly-funded research.

Universal healthcare systems invest heavily in research. Germany, UK, France, Japan, Canada—all have robust medical research. Innovation doesn't require profit-driven healthcare. It requires investment in research, which governments can fund more efficiently than extracting profits from sick people.

Patient satisfaction:

Citizens of universal healthcare countries report high satisfaction with their systems. Canadians overwhelmingly support their system despite propaganda from American politicians claiming Canadians hate it. Europeans rate their healthcare highly. Nobody's trying to copy the American model.

Meanwhile, Americans report significant dissatisfaction: insurance denials, unexpected bills, difficulty accessing care, medical debt. The most expensive system in the world generates massive frustration.

Quality requires access:

Healthcare quality isn't just clinical excellence. It's whether people can actually access care. The U.S. has 28 million uninsured people. Millions more underinsured with such high deductibles they avoid care. Excellent healthcare that's unaffordable or inaccessible isn't quality care.

Universal systems ensure everyone can access care when needed. No financial barriers. No insurance denials. No medical bankruptcy. That's quality—comprehensive access plus good clinical care.

What "best healthcare in the world" actually means:

Americans saying "we have the best healthcare" are revealing that they've never experienced healthcare in other countries. The best healthcare means:

- Everyone can access care without financial barriers
- Preventive care keeps people healthy
- Chronic disease is well-managed
- Outcomes are excellent across the population
- Nobody goes bankrupt from medical bills
- Nobody delays care due to cost

- Nobody dies from preventable conditions

By these measures, the U.S. doesn't have the best healthcare. We're not even close. We're 35th on Healthcare Access and Quality Index. We have worse outcomes and higher costs than every peer nation.

The quality objection ignores reality. Universal healthcare countries achieve better outcomes at lower cost. That's higher quality by any reasonable definition. Americans claiming quality superiority are mistaking expensive acute care for overall system performance—and losing three years of life expectancy in the process.

Why We Don't Have It: Follow the Money

Universal healthcare works everywhere it's tried. Americans support it in polling when not subjected to industry propaganda. The evidence is overwhelming that universal systems cost less and achieve better outcomes.

So why don't we have it?

Follow the money.

Healthcare industry profits:

The healthcare industry extracts enormous profits from the current system. Universal healthcare would eliminate most of those profits. The industry fights viciously to prevent reform.

While comprehensive profit data wasn't provided in research materials, lobbying expenditures reveal industry priorities:

- 2020 total healthcare lobbying: $713.6 million

- Pharmaceutical and health product manufacturers: $308.4 million
- Healthcare providers: $286.9 million
- Insurance companies: $80.6 million
- 2000-2020 increase: 70% growth in lobbying spending

From 1999-2018, the pharmaceutical and health product industry alone spent $4.7 billion on federal lobbying—an average of $233 million annually. More than any other industry.

This is spending to prevent reform. To block universal healthcare. To preserve profit extraction from illness.

Campaign contributions:

From 1999-2018, the pharmaceutical industry spent $414 million on contributions to presidential and congressional candidates, national party committees, and outside spending groups. Additionally, $877 million to state candidates and committees.

Of the 20 senators and 20 representatives receiving the most contributions, 39 belonged to committees with jurisdiction over health-related legislation, with 24 in senior positions. The industry targets politicians who control healthcare policy.

In years with state referenda on drug pricing reforms, massive spikes in contributions to groups opposing reforms. When voters tried to control drug prices through ballot initiatives, the pharmaceutical industry flooded money into defeating them.

Why the industry opposes universal healthcare

Insurance companies: Universal single-payer eliminates their business model entirely. Multi-payer universal systems heavily regulate them, capping profits. Either way, insurance industry loses revenue and power. They employ 500,000+ people in claims denial, billing, administration—jobs that would be eliminated under streamlined universal coverage.

Pharmaceutical companies: Universal systems negotiate drug prices nationally. Other countries pay half what Americans pay for identical medications. Universal healthcare in the U.S. would implement similar negotiation, cutting pharmaceutical profits dramatically.

Hospital corporations: Universal systems control reimbursement rates. Hospitals couldn't charge unlimited amounts or pursue aggressive billing. Profit margins would shrink. Private equity firms extracting wealth from hospitals would lose their investment vehicle.

Medical specialists: Fee-for-service rewards procedures over prevention, specialists over primary care. Universal systems often shift payment to value-based models, reducing specialist income while increasing primary care compensation. Specialists have opposed universal healthcare to preserve income.

Political capture:

Healthcare industry money buys political opposition to reform:

- Campaign contributions to politicians who oppose universal healthcare

- Lobbying to kill reform legislation

- Revolving door between government and industry (politicians become industry executives, industry executives appointed to government positions)

- Funding front groups claiming to represent patients or doctors but actually serving industry interests

- Running propaganda campaigns convincing voters that universal healthcare would be harmful

This political capture explains why Congress doesn't implement universal healthcare despite majority public support and overwhelming evidence it would improve outcomes while reducing costs.

Public opinion manipulation:

When asked if they support "universal healthcare" or "Medicare for All," Americans show majority or near-majority support. When the same question includes language like "government-run" or "eliminating private insurance," support drops.

The industry spends billions on propaganda convincing Americans that universal healthcare means:

- Government bureaucracy (ignoring that private insurance is more bureaucratic)

- Loss of choice (ignoring that Americans have less choice than universal systems)

- Long wait times (ignoring financial wait times Americans currently experience)

- Poor quality (ignoring that U.S. has worse outcomes than universal systems)

- Unaffordable cost (ignoring that universal healthcare costs half as much)

Every objection we've addressed in this chapter—bureaucracy, choice, wait times, quality, cost—is industry propaganda designed to prevent reform that would threaten profits.

The real reason:

We don't have universal healthcare because the current system is too profitable for too many powerful interests. Insurance companies, pharmaceutical companies, hospital corporations, private equity firms—all extract enormous wealth from healthcare. Universal healthcare would eliminate or dramatically reduce that wealth extraction.

They lobby to prevent it. They fund politicians who oppose it. They run propaganda campaigns against it. They capture the political process to prevent reform.

This isn't complicated. It's not about whether universal healthcare works—it obviously does, everywhere else proves it. It's about power and profit. The entities profiting from illness have more political power than patients dying from lack of care.

The path to universal healthcare requires overcoming that power. It requires organizing to match industry lobbying. It requires electing politicians who prioritize people over profits. It requires countering propaganda with education about how universal systems actually work.

The obstacle isn't technical or economic. It's political. We know how to implement universal healthcare. We know it would work. We're choosing not to because industry profits are prioritized over people's lives.

The Path Forward: What It Takes

Universal healthcare is achievable. Not theoretical. Not utopian. Achievable within several years if we generate the political will.

Multiple paths exist

Medicare for All (single-payer): Expand existing Medicare program to cover everyone. Most direct path. Eliminates insurance industry, maximizes administrative savings, provides comprehensive universal coverage immediately.

Could be phased in by age groups—lower Medicare eligibility age incrementally until everyone's covered—or implemented all at once. Transition period would allow insurance industry workers to find other employment, potentially with job training funded by administrative savings.

Financing through progressive income tax, eliminating regressive insurance premiums. Most families would pay less than they currently pay for insurance. Employers would save money eliminating health benefits administration.

Drug price negotiation would begin immediately, saving $100+ billion annually. Administrative savings of $375+ billion annually would more than fund expanded coverage.

Public option (compromise path): Create government insurance anyone can buy, competing with private insurance. Over time, public option becomes dominant because it's cheaper and better. Eventually the system evolves toward single-payer as private insurance loses market share.

This is less disruptive politically. It preserves private insurance initially while demonstrating government insurance superiority, and allows gradual transition rather than immediate elimination of the private insurance industry.

Regulated multi-payer (least disruptive): Mandate universal coverage with heavily regulated private insurance. Model after Germany or Switzerland: everyone required to have coverage, insurance heavily regulated (non-profit, income-based premiums, comprehensive coverage requirements, no denials), government enforces price controls.

This preserves the insurance industry while eliminating profit extraction. It requires strong sustained regulation, and is more administratively complex than single-payer, but politically easier to implement.

State-level implementation: Individual states could implement universal coverage. California has explored this. Challenges include federal cooperation requirements, interstate commerce issues, tax policy complications.

This would prove a model for national expansion. Success at state level would build momentum for federal implementation. Failure would provide lessons for improving approach.

Political requirements for any path

Overcome industry lobbying through grassroots organizing: Healthcare industry will fight viciously. Overcoming that opposition requires massive grassroots movement demanding reform. Union organizing, community organizing, patient advocacy groups building power to match industry money.

Elect politicians who prioritize people over profits: Primary and general elections must focus on healthcare. Elect representatives who refuse industry money and commit to universal coverage. Vote out politicians beholden to insurance and pharmaceutical industries.

Counter propaganda with education: Most Americans don't understand how universal healthcare works. They believe industry propaganda about government bureaucracy, loss of choice, poor quality. Education campaigns must explain reality: universal systems have less bureaucracy, more choice, better outcomes, lower costs.

Build a broad coalition: Labor unions (healthcare costs hurt workers and employers), healthcare providers (frustrated with insurance bureaucracy), patients (everyone experiences healthcare dysfunction), business owners (especially small businesses crushed by insurance costs), faith communities (healthcare as moral issue).

The coalition must be broad enough to overcome industry opposition and sustained enough to force political change.

Timeline for implementation:

Could implement within 2-4 years if political will exists. Other countries transitioned in similar timeframes. Technical challenges are solvable—we already have Medicare infrastructure that could scale. Provider networks exist. Administrative systems could be simplified dramatically.

The only obstacle is political opposition. Generate sufficient political pressure and universal healthcare could be implemented quickly.

The Transition: How We Actually Get There

The question isn't whether universal healthcare is possible. Every other wealthy nation has figured it out. The question is how we get from here to there—and whether Americans will finally demand what the rest of the developed world takes for granted.

The Legislative Landscape

Medicare for All legislation has been introduced in Congress repeatedly. The most comprehensive proposals call for a single public plan covering every American for all medically necessary services—including long-term care, mental health, dental, and prescription drugs. No premiums. No deductibles. No copays—or minimal cost-sharing that doesn't create barriers to care.

A systematic review of 22 economic analyses found that 19 of them—86%—predicted net savings in the first year of operation. The median savings: 3.46% of total costs. The largest source of savings? Simplified payment administration, which alone would save a median of 8.8%.

The evidence is overwhelming. Medicare for All would save money while covering everyone.

Medicare for All isn't the only path forward, though. Incremental approaches include offering a public option to people buying marketplace coverage, creating a Medicare or Medicaid buy-in program, lowering the Medicare eligibility age from 65 to 60 or 55 or 50, or developing a public plan that serves as the default for anyone who doesn't actively choose private coverage.

Polling reveals something interesting: 73% of Americans favor allowing people under 65 to buy Medicare coverage. Only 57% favor Medicare for All. Same policy, different framing. The words matter—because decades of industry propaganda have poisoned the term "Medicare for All" while leaving "Medicare" itself popular.

Americans love Medicare. They just don't realize that expanding it to everyone is Medicare for All.

The financing framework would repurpose existing public funds, redirect private healthcare spending to public spending, and implement progressive taxes to replace the regressive financing of private insurance. Instead of paying insurance companies $15,000 a year in premiums regardless of your income, you'd pay taxes based on what you earn. Wealthy people would pay more. Middle-class families would pay less. Poor families would pay little or nothing.

That's not radical. That's how every other developed nation does it.

Stage-level Experiments: Laboratories of Democracy

States have tried to lead where the federal government won't. The results are instructive—both the successes and the failures.

Vermont came closest. In 2011, Vermont enacted legislation to create the nation's first state-level single-payer healthcare system. According to estimates, after the first full year of operation, the system would produce annual savings of 25.3% compared to current state health spending, cut employer and household healthcare spending by $200 million, create 3,800 jobs, and boost the state's economic output by $100 million.

Vermont spent years planning. They conducted 64 semi-structured interviews with nearly 120 individuals representing 60 different stakeholder groups. They designed a politically viable reform package that addressed concerns and built support.

Then it stalled.

The obstacles were structural. State-based single-payer proposals face challenges that federal reform doesn't: states need federal permission via waivers to repurpose federal healthcare dollars. The federal Employee Retirement Income and Security Act (ERISA) preempts state regulation of employer-sponsored plans—meaning Vermont couldn't touch the insurance that large employers provide. State-only action in an interconnected 50-state economy creates economic disadvantages that federal reform avoids.

Vermont's failure wasn't because single-payer doesn't work. It was because states can't implement universal healthcare alone when the federal government designed the system to prevent exactly that.

California keeps trying. In 2017, the state Senate passed the Healthy California Act, calling for California to adopt single-payer. The Assembly held hearings highlighting both the benefits and the challenges—including the need for federal cooperation and new state taxes to replace employer and employee insurance payments.

California's single-payer legislation is stalled, but the state established a task force to pursue unified public financing. The conversation continues.

The most likely result of state-level efforts? Incremental public insurance expansions—programs letting uninsured people buy into Medicaid, public options competing with private insurance, coverage expansions for specific populations. Not true single-payer, but steps toward universal coverage.

Incrementalism. It's not what we need, but it may be the path we take—because the federal government refuses to act and states are doing what they can within the constraints of a system designed to prevent reform.

Timeline Scenarios: How Fast Could This Happen?

History offers two models: rapid transformation and gradual expansion.

The Rapid Path: Taiwan

Taiwan implemented universal single-payer national health insurance in 1995. Coverage expanded from 57% of the population to 98% essentially overnight.

On its twentieth anniversary in 2015, Taiwan's National Health Insurance stood out as a high-performing system providing universal coverage to 23.4 million residents based on egalitarian ethical principles, delivering affordable modern healthcare without the waiting times seen in systems like England and Canada.

Taiwan's experience proves that single-payer can work and control costs effectively. But here's the critical piece: Taiwan spent two decades preparing. They built up healthcare infrastructure—hospitals, clinics, trained providers—before implementing universal coverage. They used tax incentives and subsidies to enhance public-private partnerships. They addressed regional disparities through incentives and regulation. They safeguarded quality through licensing and accreditation. They promoted evidence-based policymaking.

The lesson: rapid implementation is possible, but requires extensive preparation. You can't expand coverage to 98% of the population overnight if you don't have the infrastructure to actually provide care to 98% of the population.

The Gradual Path: Canada

Canada's path took decades.

In 1947, Saskatchewan became the first jurisdiction with universal health coverage in North America, initially covering hospital care only. In 1962, Saskatchewan expanded to medical care—prompting a doctors' strike that lasted 23 days. The strike ended with the Saskatoon Agreement establishing opt-out provisions and protections for fee-for-service private practice.

Sound familiar? Doctors threatening to strike rather than participate in universal coverage. Industry propaganda about government control. Dire predictions of rationing and poor quality.

The doctors were wrong then. They're wrong now.

The federal government encouraged other provinces to adopt the Saskatchewan approach by offering 50 cents for every provincial dollar spent on universal coverage. By 1958, five provinces were participating in hospital insurance. By 1961, all ten provinces had joined. The Medical Care Insurance Act passed Parliament in 1966 and came into effect in 1968. By 1971, all provinces had established comprehensive medical insurance plans meeting federal criteria.

The process culminated in 1984 with the unanimous adoption of the Canada Health Act, which explicitly banned extra billing and established criteria for transfer payment eligibility: public administration, comprehensiveness, universality, portability, and accessibility.

Total timeline: roughly 37 years from Saskatchewan's first hospital insurance to the Canada Health Act. But the core expansion—from one province to all provinces covering both hospital and medical care—took about 24 years.

Not overnight, but nonetheless inevitable, once it started.

The UK's Post-War Transformation

The UK's National Health Service was created in 1948, emerging from World War II when the central government had established an Emergency Medical Service to oversee hospitals during the war. The Beveridge Report set out the blueprint for a universal welfare state.

Minister of Health Aneurin Bevan had a bold vision: comprehensive medical services as a universal right, free at the point of use, funded predominantly from progressive taxation, with hospitals nationalized under a unitary system.

The British Medical Association organized a plebiscite of members to demonstrate their refusal to participate. Medical correspondents aired negative comments against the purported "gigantic bureaucratic machine" and warned of "totalitarianism."

Sound familiar?

Despite opposition, the NHS was implemented in approximately two years from legislation to operation. July 5, 1948—the "appointed day"—hospitals throughout Britain were incorporated into this vast enterprise. Since then, healthcare in the United Kingdom has been centrally funded through the NHS, providing both primary and specialist healthcare largely free at the point of delivery.

The doctors predicted disaster. They got the most popular institution in British society instead.

What History Teaches Us

Countries are achieving universal coverage faster now than in the past. Malaysia and South Korea reached universal health coverage in two to three decades at lower income levels than the higher-income countries that preceded them. The learning curve has shortened as countries study previous successes and failures.

We know what works. We know what doesn't. We have seventy-five years of international experience to draw from—successes to replicate, mistakes to avoid.

The question isn't "Can we do this?" The question is "Will we?"

Phase-in Approaches: Who Gets Covered First?

Universal health coverage has historically been achieved incrementally, with different population subgroups incorporated gradually. In systems relying on social insurance, coverage typically began with employees of large firms, followed by small firms, rural workers, the self-employed, and eventually the unemployed and indigent.

The United States could follow several phase-in approaches.

By Age: Lower the Medicare eligibility age incrementally—from 65 to 60, then 55, then 50—until everyone is covered. This builds on existing infrastructure and public familiarity with Medicare. It's politically easier because it expands a popular program rather than creating something new.

Research shows that entry into Medicare at age 65 increases access to care and improves health for people previously without insurance, with reductions in racial and ethnic disparities in access. Expanding Medicare downward would extend those benefits to younger populations.

By Income: Expand Medicaid and marketplace subsidies to cover lower-income populations first, then gradually raise income thresholds. Mexico used this approach with its Seguro Popular program, focusing on poor and marginalized groups ineligible for employment-based insurance.

The challenge with income-based phase-ins: they risk creating a two-tier system where wealthier people have private insurance and poorer people have public insurance. That's politically vulnerable—because when only poor people depend on a program, funding that program becomes less popular.

Universal programs—Medicare, Social Security—are politically untouchable because everyone benefits. Means-tested programs—Medicaid, food stamps—face constant attacks because only poor people benefit and poor people have less political power.

All at Once: Taiwan's approach—comprehensive implementation after extensive preparation. Everyone covered from day one. This avoids the political vulnerability of partial programs and ensures everyone has a stake in the system's success immediately.

The American College of Physicians has outlined two potential approaches: a single-payer model and a public choice model. The public choice model would maintain existing coverage options while adding a robust public plan—potentially serving as a transition mechanism toward single-payer as people voluntarily choose the public option and private insurance loses market share.

There's no perfect approach, but any of these paths would be better than what we have now.

The Role of Existing Medicare Infrastructure

Medicare already covers more than 55 million Americans—most aged 65 or older, plus 9 million younger adults with permanent disabilities. Together, Medicare and Medicaid provide health coverage to about 111 million people—one in three Americans.

The infrastructure exists.

Medicare's administrative costs are 1.35% of benefits—compared to 10.86-14.84% for Medicare Advantage plans run by private insurance companies, and 15-20% for private insurance generally. The program already processes billions of claims annually, negotiates with providers, and maintains quality standards.

Scaling Medicare to cover everyone would require addressing several implementation challenges. Provider payment rates would need adjustment—Medicare pays hospitals and doctors less than private insurance does, so if everyone suddenly had Medicare, providers would see revenue decreases unless reimbursement rates increased. Utilization would increase as newly covered populations accessed care they'd been avoiding. Enrollment systems would need expansion.

But the fundamental infrastructure already exists: claims processing systems, provider networks, quality oversight mechanisms, fraud detection, and appeals processes—all of it operates right now for 55 million people. Scaling to 330 million people is a technical challenge, not a conceptual one.

Under single-payer, physicians would have multiple payment options: fee-for-service with a simple binding fee schedule, salaried practice in institutions receiving global budgets, or salaried practice in capitated group practices. Billing would be simplified—physicians would submit bills on a simple form or via computer and receive payment within 30 days, with interest for bills not paid on time.

No prior authorization fights. No claim denials. No checking whether patients have met their deductibles. No network restrictions. Just healthcare.

What Happens to Insurance Industry Workers?

This is the question that haunts every serious discussion of healthcare reform—and it's a legitimate concern.

National health insurance would eliminate many administrative and insurance worker positions. Not all of them—Medicare still needs administrators, claims processors, customer service representatives. The massive bureaucracies that private insurance companies employ on the other hand, the staff needed to deny claims, fight appeals, determine network coverage, and maximize revenue while minimizing payouts? Those jobs would disappear.

That's hundreds of thousands of people whose livelihoods depend on the current system.

The Physicians' Working Group proposal suggests that many displaced workers might be redeployed as support personnel to free up nurses for clinical tasks. Others might be retrained to staff expanded programs in public health, home care, and similar services. Hospitals' administrative departments would shrink, but clinical departments would see only modest changes beyond the elimination of billing-related work.

The transition would need to include:

- Severance and income support during the transition period
- Retraining programs for healthcare administration, public health, and clinical support roles
- Early retirement options for older workers
- Hiring preferences in the new system for displaced workers

The hundreds of billions saved annually on insurance-related bureaucracy could fund generous transition support while still achieving net savings. A portion of the $375-471 billion in administrative waste we currently spend could go toward retraining and supporting displaced workers, and we'd still save hundreds of billions.

The question is political will, not economic feasibility.

Here's what I want you to understand: I have empathy for insurance industry workers. Most of them are just people trying to make a living, pay their bills, and support their families. They didn't design this system. They're not responsible for its cruelty.

That said, the industry employs them specifically to create barriers to care. Their jobs exist to deny claims, fight appeals, restrict access, and maximize insurance company profits by minimizing payouts to patients. That's not their fault—it's the fault of a system designed to profit from denying care.

We can transition those workers to other roles. We can provide generous support. We can retrain and redeploy them into positions that actually help people rather than positions that exist to deny them care.

What we can't do is let hundreds of thousands of jobs that shouldn't exist prevent us from building a healthcare system that actually works.

Global Budgets And Payment Reform

Single-payer proposals typically include global budgeting for hospitals—setting an overall budget for the year rather than paying per service. This changes incentives fundamentally.

Taiwan adopted system-wide global budgets to control healthcare expenditure growth, setting a hard aggregate budget cap to limit total spending to expected revenue, with annual growth rates established through negotiation among key stakeholders.

An economic analysis estimated that non-federal hospital operating budgets would total $17.2 trillion between 2021 and 2030 under current law versus $14.7 trillion under single-payer with global budgets—reflecting $520 billion in foregone profits and $1,984 billion in reduced administrative expenditures.

Think about that. Under current law, hospitals would spend $17.2 trillion. Under single-payer, they'd spend $14.7 trillion and provide the same care to more people. The difference—$2.5 trillion—is profit extraction and administrative waste.

Global budgets change incentives. Operating revenues become stable and predictable. Capital requests are weighed against other priorities for healthcare investment. Facilities don't grow or shrink based on financial performance—they grow or shrink based on health needs.

Some hospitals would need to expand. Others would need to close—particularly the ones that exist only because they're profitable, not because the community needs them. That's rational health planning. That's treating healthcare as a public good rather than a profit center.

The Political Reality

Movement toward universal health coverage is a long-term policy engagement that needs both technical knowledge and political know-how. Technical solutions need to be accompanied by pragmatic and innovative strategies that address the national political economy context.

Translation: knowing the right policy isn't enough. You have to overcome the political power of the entities profiting from the current system.

The institutions created to provide universal health coverage are negotiated rather than designed—they're the outcomes of politics and contestation. The UK's National Health Service was originally planned to be financed with payroll taxes, but demand grew quickly and governments chose to rely increasingly on general revenues. Political processes alter health system designs in unpredictable ways.

What's required is persistent social pressure, widespread public demand, and ultimately government action despite opposition from vested interests.

The largest expansion of public health coverage in the United States occurred in the 1960s when the government overcame opposition from groups including the American Medical Association to create Medicare and Medicaid. Industry opposition was fierce. Predictions of disaster were dire. The AMA called Medicare "socialized medicine" that would destroy American healthcare.

They were wrong. Medicare became one of the most popular and successful government programs in American history.

Political winds can shift. The transition from Hoover's aversion to social spending to Roosevelt's New Deal took just a few years. The Civil Rights and Great Society advances followed the McCarthy era. Healthcare destabilization and public backlash against broken promises can open unforeseen options for reform.

We're in a moment of healthcare destabilization right now. The Thompson assassination revealed collective rage at system cruelty. Medical bankruptcy continues destroying families. People are dying from lack of insurance. The current system is unsustainable both economically and morally.

That creates opportunities for change—if we're organized enough to seize them.

The Bottom Line

A single-payer universal healthcare system would save more than 68,000 lives and 1.73 million life-years every year compared with the status quo. The entire system could be funded with less financial outlay than is currently incurred by employers and households paying for healthcare premiums combined with existing government allocations.

Read that again: universal healthcare covering everyone would cost less than what we're already paying.

The transition is feasible. Other countries have done it—some rapidly, some gradually, all successfully. The infrastructure exists. The financing works. The savings are real.

What's missing is political will.

And political will is a choice.

Every year we delay, 68,000 more Americans die who didn't have to. Every year we delay, 530,000 more families face medical bankruptcy. Every year we delay, we spend hundreds of billions more on administrative waste that could be funding actual healthcare.

The path forward exists. We just have to decide to take it.

The question isn't "Can we afford universal healthcare?" We're already paying for it twice over.

The question is: "Are we willing to build it?"

What Would My Work Be Like Under Universal Healthcare?

I envision treating patients without insurance company interference. No prior authorization fights. No claim denials to appeal. No patients avoiding care because they can't afford it. Just healthcare.

Patients wouldn't worry about bills. They'd come in when sick rather than waiting until conditions become emergencies. I wouldn't see the December rush of patients trying to "get free healthcare" because they met their deductible before the end of year—that desperate behavior revealing how broken the current system is.

We'd be busier, most definitely.. More people accessing care they currently avoid due to cost. That's good, though. People need care. Universal healthcare would let them get it.

Maybe we'd need more providers. Maybe medical school would be funded or incentivized—free tuition in exchange for service, loan forgiveness, higher compensation for primary care to attract more doctors. Universal systems can afford this because administrative savings would be enormous.

The preventive care we'd provide would save lives. People wouldn't wait until diabetes causes kidney failure or heart attacks require emergency intervention. They'd get routine care, catch problems early, manage conditions before complications develop.

Every person who's been scared to see a doctor because of cost would benefit. We'd save lives through prevention—exactly what healthcare is supposed to do.

This isn't fantasy. This is how healthcare works everywhere else. Providers focus on medicine. Patients access care without financial terror. Systems invest in health rather than profit extraction.

I want this. I want to do my job without insurance companies deciding what care my patients can receive. I want patients to focus on healing rather than bankruptcy. I want American healthcare to function like healthcare instead of a profit-driven industry.

Why I Want Universal Healthcare

I want the United States to value and care for its citizens the way every other developed nation does. I want healthcare to be a right, not something people beg for on GoFundMe or avoid until they're dying because they can't afford it.

I want people to have money in their pockets because they're not spending $1,000 monthly on insurance premiums only to be denied coverage when they actually need care. I want families to stop going bankrupt from medical bills. I want the 530,000 families currently bankrupted annually by healthcare costs to keep their homes and savings.

I want uninsured people to see providers without fear. I want the 28 million Americans currently uninsured to have comprehensive coverage automatically. I want the 68,000 Americans who die annually from lack of insurance to live.

I'm tired of patients rationing medications because they can't afford them. I'm tired of watching people deteriorate from preventable conditions because they couldn't access care early. I'm tired of fighting insurance companies over coverage that should be automatic. I'm tired of the system being designed to extract profit from suffering rather than promote health.

I'm tired of pretending American healthcare is acceptable when every other developed nation proves better systems exist.

This book exists because Americans need to understand: our healthcare system is sick by design.

Designed to maximize profit, not health.

Designed to deny care while collecting premiums.

Designed to keep people dependent on employers rather than enabling economic freedom.

Designed to benefit corporations at the expense of patients.

Universal healthcare would fix this. Cover everyone. Control costs. Eliminate medical bankruptcy. Focus on health rather than profit. Save tens of thousands of lives annually while saving hundreds of billions in costs.

The path exists. The evidence is overwhelming. The only question is whether we'll choose it.

Hope vs. Cynicism

Will we actually get universal healthcare? I think we might. Not sure it will be in my lifetime. Maybe in my daughters' lifetime.

The political obstacles are substantial. Healthcare industry opposition is fierce. Propaganda is effective. Americans have been convinced that universal healthcare would be harmful despite all evidence to the contrary.

Meanwhile, conditions are deteriorating. Healthcare costs keep rising. Medical bankruptcy continues destroying families. People keep dying from preventable causes. The current system is unsustainable economically and morally.

At some point, Americans will demand change. Healthcare destabilization creates opportunities for reform. When enough people experience the system's cruelty directly—denied care, medical bankruptcy, loved ones dying from preventable conditions—they become willing to fight for alternatives.

The COVID-19 pandemic demonstrated system failures. Millions lost employer-based insurance during the worst possible time. People avoided care due to cost, worsening outcomes. The pandemic killed an estimated 212,000 additional Americans due to lack of universal coverage—deaths that wouldn't have occurred in countries with universal healthcare.

That kind of crisis creates political will for change. Not immediately—industry opposition remains powerful. Gradually, though, Americans are recognizing that the current system isn't working. Support for universal healthcare has grown, particularly among younger Americans who've never known affordable, accessible healthcare.

I'm cautiously hopeful. Not optimistic that change is imminent, but hopeful that it's possible. The evidence is too clear, the failures too widespread, the suffering too extensive. Eventually, Americans will demand better.

The alternative is continuing to accept that American healthcare bankrupts families, kills people, costs twice as much as peer nations while achieving worse outcomes. Keep accepting that our children will face the same broken system we've endured. Keep accepting that profit matters more than health.

I don't think Americans will accept that forever. Change is coming. Slowly, against massive opposition, but coming.

Whether I see it in my lifetime, or my daughter does—it's coming. Because the current system is unsustainable and universal healthcare is the obvious solution. Industry can delay it, but they can't prevent it indefinitely.

You Deserve Better

Keep pressing forward. Vote for politicians who support universal healthcare. Don't think of universal healthcare as charity or handout. It's how civilized nations treat healthcare—as a right, not a commodity.

You deserve healthcare without bankruptcy. You deserve to see doctors without financial terror. You deserve a system that keeps you healthy rather than profiting from your illness.

Universal healthcare isn't radical. It's standard in the developed world. Every peer nation has it. All achieve better outcomes at lower cost. It works. It's proven. It's not some theoretical experiment—it's reality in Canada, UK, France, Germany, Japan, Australia, and everywhere else that decided health matters more than profit.

Don't let propaganda convince you that universal healthcare means poor quality or restricted access. Americans already have restricted access—through insurance networks, prior authorization, claim denials, unaffordable costs. Universal systems provide more access, better outcomes, less bureaucracy.

Don't let industry claims about unaffordable costs convince you it's impossible. We're already paying twice as much as countries with universal coverage. We're spending enough to fund comprehensive universal healthcare for everyone. The money's there—it's just going to corporate profits instead of patient care.

Don't accept that medical bankruptcy is normal. It's uniquely American. It doesn't happen in other developed countries. It's not inevitable—it's a policy choice we could change.

Don't believe you have to choose between a job you hate and losing healthcare. Employer-based insurance is an accident of history, not an inevitable feature of healthcare. Other countries separated healthcare from employment decades ago. You could start a business, change careers, work part-time—without risking healthcare access.

Universal healthcare is achievable. Other countries prove it daily. We can have it, too.

It requires demanding it, voting for it, organizing for it. It requires refusing to accept industry propaganda, and building political power to overcome industry opposition.

It requires believing Americans deserve what every other developed nation provides: healthcare as a right, comprehensive coverage for all residents, no financial barriers to care, no medical bankruptcy, no deaths from lack of insurance.

You deserve this. Your children deserve this. Future generations deserve this.

The path exists. The question is whether we'll take it.

Research Notes:

This chapter synthesizes international healthcare system comparisons documenting that universal coverage models (single-payer like Canada, heavily regulated multi-payer like Germany/France, and hybrid systems like Australia) all achieve better health outcomes at approximately half the per capita cost of the U.S. system. Wait time data shows the U.S. at 6% waiting 2+ months for specialists compared to 3-9% in European multi-payer systems and higher rates in Canada (39%) and UK (19%), with emergency care immediate in all systems. Administrative cost data reveals U.S. spending 34.2% of healthcare expenditures ($812 billion annually) on administration versus 17.0% in Canada and 1-3% for single-payer government insurance, with Medicare overhead at 1.35% versus private insurance at 15-20%. Multiple cost analyses project Medicare for All would save $300-600 billion annually through administrative efficiency and negotiated drug prices. Healthcare industry lobbying totaled $713.6 million in 2020 (70% increase from 2000), with the pharmaceutical industry spending $4.7 billion on federal lobbying from 1999-2018. Studies estimate universal healthcare would save 68,000+ American lives annually, with 212,000 preventable COVID-19 deaths attributable to lack of universal coverage. Personal perspectives integrate clinical experience with insurance-based barriers to care and vision for a healthcare system focused on health rather than profit extraction.

Conclusion: Choosing Health Over Profit

I started this book with Brian Thompson's assassination because that moment revealed something America had been trying to ignore: millions of people understand why someone would kill a healthcare CEO.

Not justify it. Not celebrate it. *Understand* it.

In Chapter 8, we examined what Thompson's assassination revealed about our healthcare system—the denial rates, the bullet casings etched with "deny, defend, depose," the collective rage expressed through memes instead of mourning. As we close this book, though, I need to be honest about what that moment revealed about me.

When I heard a healthcare CEO had been killed, I felt no empathy for him. I'm ashamed of that. Violence is never the answer, and a man died leaving behind people who loved him.

That said, I still understood why millions of Americans felt what I felt at that moment: exhausted recognition that the system Thompson represented kills people every single day through legal, profitable, designed-in cruelty—and nobody faces consequences for those deaths because they generate profit for corporations and campaign donations for politicians.

The question Americans asked in the assassinations aftermath was uncomfortable but unavoidable: Why should we show empathy for people profiting from our suffering?

Insurance companies show no empathy when they deny coverage for cancer treatment.

Pharmaceutical companies show no empathy when they price insulin at $300 per vial.

Hospital corporations show no empathy when they sue patients into bankruptcy.

Politicians show no empathy when they take insurance company donations and block reform.

The answer to that question matters less than what we do next. Because here's the uncomfortable truth: Brian Thompson's assassination changes nothing unless we make it change something.

UnitedHealthcare still denies claims. Pharmaceutical companies still price-gouge. Hospitals still sue patients. Insurance companies still lobby politicians to prevent reform. The system that created the rage that led to Thompson's murder continues operating exactly as before.

One CEO dies. Another takes his place. The machine keeps running.

Unless we choose to stop it.

The Design, Piece by Piece

That's the choice this book has been documenting: a healthcare system designed to extract maximum profit from human suffering.

We built healthcare on racist exclusions. The Social Security Act of 1935 deliberately excluded agricultural workers and domestic servants—the occupations that employed two-thirds of Black Americans—ensuring that government benefits would primarily serve white workers.

The Hill-Burton Act of 1946 funded "separate but equal" hospital construction, cementing segregation into healthcare infrastructure. Every foundation of American healthcare was designed to serve some people while excluding others.

We tied healthcare to employment, not by rational policy design but by wartime accident that became permanent because it served corporate interests. Employer-based insurance gave companies leverage over workers, created job lock that restricted economic mobility, and ensured that losing your job meant losing healthcare exactly when you needed it most. This wasn't a bug. It was a feature that kept workers dependent.

We let pharmaceutical companies write their own rules. Patent manipulation, pay-for-delay deals, government-funded research privatized for profit, regulatory capture that blocks price negotiation, lobbying expenditures exceeding $4.7 billion from 1999 to 2018—the opioid crisis alone killed hundreds of thousands of Americans because the Sackler family and Purdue Pharma designed OxyContin's marketing to maximize addiction and profit. Drug prices aren't high because of research costs. They're high because we chose to let pharmaceutical companies charge whatever they want.

We built a reactive system that profits from treating illness rather than preventing it. Fee-for-service payment rewards volume over value, insurance churn means companies don't benefit from prevention, and primary care physicians earn half what specialists make despite being the foundation of health. The system isn't failing to prevent disease—it's succeeding at maximizing revenue from treating disease after it develops.

We weaponized preexisting conditions. Before the ACA, insurance companies denied coverage, excluded conditions, charged unaffordable premiums, and practiced rescission—waiting until people got sick to cancel their policies based on technicalities. Even after the ACA banned the most egregious practices, the system still functions to screen out expensive patients, restrict access through narrow networks, and shift costs to individuals through deductibles that make insurance meaningless until you've already spent thousands.

We normalized medical bankruptcy. 530,000 American families file bankruptcy due to medical bills annually—even when they have insurance. Medical debt totals $88 billion in collections. Hospitals sue patients for unpaid bills, garnish wages, place liens on homes. This isn't an unfortunate side effect of an otherwise functional system. This is the system working exactly as designed: transferring healthcare costs to individuals while extracting maximum profit for corporations.

We created the entrepreneur's trap. Starting a business means losing employer-based insurance, facing marketplace premiums of $650-1,130 per month with $6,500-7,500+ deductibles, navigating coverage cliffs where earning $1 more can cost you thousands in subsidies. The system deliberately discourages entrepreneurship by making healthcare contingent on traditional employment.

Every piece of dysfunction is intentional. Every piece serves profit. Every piece harms patients while enriching corporations.

The Choice We Face

So what are you going to do about it?

You can accept it. Go back to your life, your job, your employer-based insurance—if you have it. Hope you don't get sick. Hope your insurance doesn't deny claims. Hope medical bills don't bankrupt you. Hope is free. It's also useless when the system is designed to fail you.

Or you can fight it.

Every other developed nation chose to fight it. They built universal healthcare systems that cover everyone, cost half as much as American healthcare, and achieve better outcomes. Canada, the UK, France, Germany, Japan, Australia, Taiwan, South Korea—different models, different structures, but all sharing core principles:

- Everyone is covered.
- Coverage is based on residency, not employment.
- Prices are regulated to prevent profit extraction.
- Financial barriers to care are eliminated.
- Prevention is prioritized over treatment.
- Administrative costs are minimal.
- Medical bankruptcy doesn't exist.

These aren't theoretical systems. They're real, they work, and they've worked for decades. The evidence is overwhelming. The only question is whether Americans will demand them.

What You Can Do Right Now

You've read the evidence. You understand the system. You know that 68,000 Americans die every year because we chose profit over people.

The question now is: what are you going to do about it?

Universal healthcare won't happen because politicians suddenly develop consciences. It will happen because ordinary people make it politically impossible to maintain the status quo. Every major expansion of healthcare coverage in American history—Medicare, Medicaid, the ACA—came from sustained social pressure that made inaction more costly than action.

This isn't a chapter about feeling good. This is your toolkit for actually changing things.

Understand The Political Reality

First, consider this truth: universal health coverage is fundamentally a political challenge, not a technical one.

The evidence for universal coverage is overwhelming. The economics work. Other countries have done it successfully for decades. The barrier isn't knowledge—it's power.

The healthcare industry spends over $700 million annually on lobbying because they understand this. They know that political power, not policy papers, determines outcomes. They know that the best-designed policy proposal in the world means nothing if you can't overcome the political opposition of entities making hundreds of billions in profits from the current system.

Your job is to build countervailing power.

Advocates for universal health coverage must understand that achieving it reflects the contestation of political interests, prevailing ideas and beliefs, and decisions mediated through political institutions. That's academic language for: this is a fight. You're fighting insurance companies, pharmaceutical companies, hospital corporations, and every politician who takes their money.

They have money. You have numbers—if you organize.

Join Organizations That Are Actually Fighting

Not all healthcare advocacy organizations are created equal. Some are genuinely fighting for universal coverage. Others are industry-funded fronts that exist to channel legitimate anger into ineffective action.

Here's something that should enrage you: two-thirds of patient advocacy organizations receive industry funding. Some receive more than half their budget from pharmaceutical, device, and biotechnology companies. Organizations dependent on industry money rarely bite the hand that feeds them.

So when you're deciding which organizations to join and support, look for:

Financial independence from industry. Does the organization take pharmaceutical money? Insurance money? If they're funded by the entities profiting from the current system, they're not going to fight to change it.

Clear policy positions. Does the organization explicitly support universal coverage? Medicare for All? A robust public option? Or does it focus on incremental tweaks that leave the fundamental system intact while making donors feel like they're helping?

Track record of confrontation. Has the organization actually challenged powerful interests? Or does it specialize in "partnerships" and "stakeholder engagement" that produce glossy reports and exactly zero policy changes?

The most effective organizations combine grassroots mobilization with policy expertise. They understand that civil society exerts power by mobilizing evidence, advocating for legislation, through electoral campaigning, litigation, public education, lobbying, and political strategies intended to disrupt the status quo such as boycotts, strikes, demonstrations, and sit-ins.

Translation: they're willing to actually fight, not just write position papers.

Look for organizations that:

- Organize people, not just fundraise from them
- Have clear demands and won't settle for symbolic victories
- Build coalitions across movements—labor, civil rights, faith communities
- Understand that changing healthcare requires challenging corporate power

I'm not going to name specific organizations here because the landscape changes and I don't want this book to become outdated. Do your research. Find organizations that are actually fighting. Join them. Support them. Show up when they organize actions.

Counter The Propaganda

When you talk to family and friends about healthcare, you're not just sharing information—you're fighting a propaganda war against billions of dollars in industry messaging.

The good news: research shows that how healthcare proposals are framed dramatically affects public support.

The bad news: most people are terrible at framing because they don't understand the propaganda they're fighting against.

Here's what research shows works:

- Names matter. Including the names "Medicare For All" and "Medicaid Buy-In" increases approval by 3.4 and 5.0 percentage points respectively compared to describing the same policies without names. People trust expansions of programs they know.

- So don't say "government healthcare." Say "expanding Medicare to cover everyone." Don't say "creating a new system." Say "letting people buy into Medicaid."

- Framing as expansion works. Approval is higher for health policies framed as expansions of existing policies than as new programs. "Expanding Medicare" polls better than "creating a new government healthcare system"—even though they're the same thing.

- Public support is broader than reported. During the ACA debate, support for the public option ranged from 46.5% to 64.6% depending on how pollsters worded their questions. The "divided public" narrative often reflects biased

> question wording, not actual public opinion. When you hear that Americans are "divided" on healthcare, what you're actually hearing is that pollsters asked loaded questions designed to generate that result.

When someone repeats industry talking points, don't just argue—reframe.

They say: "Government takeover"
You say: "Expanding Medicare, the most popular insurance program in America, to cover everyone"

They say: "You'll lose your doctor"
You say: "You'll never lose coverage because you changed jobs, and you can see any doctor who accepts Medicare—which is almost all of them. Right now you lose your doctor every time your employer changes insurance companies."

They say: "It's too expensive"
You say: "We already spend twice what other countries spend. Universal coverage would save money while covering everyone. The question isn't whether we can afford universal healthcare—we're already paying for it three times over. The question is whether we're willing to stop letting insurance companies extract hundreds of billions in profits."

They say: "Long wait times"
You say: "Americans already wait—we just call it 'delaying care because we can't afford it.' Twenty-five percent of Americans skip needed care due to cost. That's the real wait time. Other countries have scheduling waits for elective procedures. We have financial waits that kill people."

The most effective corrections come from trusted sources. Healthcare professionals correcting misinformation are particularly credible. If you work in healthcare, your voice carries weight—use it.

But here's the critical piece: don't just correct misinformation. Offer the alternative frame immediately. Research shows that debunking works better when you provide the accurate information right after addressing the false claim.

Use Your Story

Personal narratives are powerful tools for policy change. Your healthcare horror story—the denied claim, the impossible bill, the coverage gap, the bankruptcy—isn't just personal suffering. It's political ammunition.

Research shows that patient narratives convey information that complements and augments epidemiological evidence, generating persuasive evidence with important potential for influencing policy and practice. Three-quarters of patient narratives contain actionable content that can drive quality improvement and policy change.

Translation: your story matters. It changes minds and influences policy—if you use it strategically.

How to use your story effectively:

- **Be specific.** Names, dates, dollar amounts, consequences. "My insurance denied my claim" is less powerful than "[Insurance Company Name] denied coverage for my daughter's chemotherapy in March 2024, claiming it wasn't medically necessary despite her oncologist's recommendation. We paid $47,000 out of pocket while fighting the appeal for six months."

- Specificity creates credibility. Details make it real.
- **Connect personal to systemic.** Your story isn't about bad luck—it's about a system designed to produce these outcomes. "This didn't happen because I had bad insurance. This happened because insurance companies profit by denying claims. My experience isn't unique—it's typical."
- **Identify the villain.** Insurance company? Hospital billing department? Pharmaceutical company? Policy that created the problem? Make the systemic cause clear. Don't let people write off your story as an unfortunate exception. Name the entity or policy that caused the harm.
- **Propose the solution.** Don't just describe the problem. Connect your story to the policy change that would prevent it from happening to others. "Under Medicare for All, this wouldn't happen. My daughter would have gotten her chemotherapy immediately without fighting an insurance company for approval."

Share your story with elected officials, at town halls, in letters to editors, on social media, with journalists covering healthcare. Tag politicians on social media when you share your story. Make them respond to you in public.

People with lived experience who share their stories can lead changes in policy and services. But you have to actually share it. Private suffering changes nothing. Public testimony creates political pressure.

Support Mutual Aid While Fighting for Systemic Change

Mutual aid—neighbors helping neighbors meet survival needs—proliferated during the COVID-19 pandemic as government failures left needs unmet. People organized GoFundMe campaigns for medical bills, prescription sharing networks, transportation to appointments, childcare during hospitalizations.
Let me be clear: mutual aid is not a solution to systemic healthcare failure.

What it is, is a survival strategy while we fight for universal coverage—and a way to build the solidarity networks that make political organizing possible.

Research on mutual aid groups found that meeting community needs with localized action, building trust and community-based alliances, and creating a culture of care and support helped sustain involvement and build lasting community cohesion. These same networks can be mobilized for political action.

So participate in mutual aid. Help your neighbors. Build community. But never let anyone tell you that GoFundMe is an acceptable healthcare system or that neighbor-helping-neighbor replaces the need for universal coverage.

Mutual aid keeps people alive while we fight for the system that should exist. It's a bandaid on a hemorrhage—necessary for survival but not a substitute for surgery.

Community health initiatives that work directly with affected communities to co-develop healthcare solutions demonstrate that the factors contributing to health can only be addressed by working in partnership with communities. Building these partnerships creates the foundation for political mobilization.

You need both: immediate mutual aid to survive the current system, and organized political action to change it.

Make Healthcare a Voting Issue

Healthcare consistently ranks among the top issues for voters. In 2018, four in ten likely voters identified healthcare as an "extremely important" issue when deciding how to vote. The top concerns: protecting coverage for preexisting conditions, lowering costs, protecting Medicare, and preventing coverage losses.

But healthcare only drives electoral outcomes when voters connect their healthcare experiences to their voting decisions—and when they actually vote.

Here's what matters: voter turnout among people who were registered to vote in healthcare settings increased from 61% in 2016 to 79.8% in 2020—a gain 7.7 percentage points higher than the general population. Healthcare professionals helped initiate over 27,000 voter registrations and 17,000 mail-in ballot requests through healthcare-based outreach in 2020.

Healthcare settings can be powerful venues for voter registration and mobilization because they reach younger and more racially diverse populations than traditional political campaigns. Physicians and nurses are trusted messengers who can encourage civic engagement.

What you can do:

- **Register to vote and verify your registration before every election.** Voter purges happen. Don't assume you're still registered—check.

- **Vote in every election.** Primaries. Local elections. School boards. Not just presidential years. Local and state officials often have more direct impact on healthcare access than federal politicians. State-level experiments can build momentum for national change.

- **Help others register and vote, especially in healthcare settings.** If you work in healthcare, you have unique access to people who are directly experiencing the consequences of our broken system. Help them register. Help them get to the polls. Provide information about candidates' healthcare positions.

- **Make healthcare your litmus test.** Don't vote for candidates who oppose universal coverage, regardless of party. I don't care what else they support. If they're taking insurance company money and opposing Medicare for All or a robust public option, they're part of the problem.

Single-issue voting gets a bad reputation, but healthcare isn't a single issue—it affects everything. Economic security, racial justice, worker rights, entrepreneurship, family stability. If a politician won't fight for universal healthcare, they're not fighting for you.

Pressure Tactics That Work

Politicians respond to pressure. The question is what kind of pressure works.

Research on civil society influence on health policy identifies several factors that enhance effectiveness: joining strong networks and broader coalitions of stakeholders, being well-resourced, and framing issues in ways that resonate with national policies and political priorities.

Translation: organize, build coalitions, and make politicians believe that opposing universal healthcare will cost them their jobs.

Effective pressure tactics:

- **Show up.** Town halls, public meetings, campaign events. Politicians notice when constituents are physically present and vocal. Congressional staff track who attends events and what issues they raise. Be that person raising healthcare at every opportunity.

- **Flood the phones.** Coordinated call campaigns to congressional offices work. Staff track call volume and topics. One constituent calling once gets noted. Fifty constituents calling the same week about the same issue gets action.

- **Build coalitions.** Healthcare reform requires alliances across labor, civil rights, faith communities, and other movements. Grassroots health care demands have contained the seeds of wider critique, leading movements to adopt calls for universal coverage.

You can't win this fight alone. Labor unions should be fighting for universal healthcare because it would free workers from job lock and strengthen their bargaining position. Civil rights organizations should be fighting for it because the current system is built on racism and perpetuates racial health disparities. Faith communities should be fighting for it because healthcare is a moral issue. Environmental groups should be fighting for it because climate change is a health crisis.

Build those alliances. Make universal healthcare a demand across movements.

- **Pressure the right politicians.** Focus pressure on elected officials in competitive districts who need your vote. A politician in a safe district can ignore you. A politician facing a competitive election can't.

- **Find out who your representatives are.** Find out whether they're vulnerable. If they are, make them feel it.

- **Make it local.** State and local officials often have more direct impact on healthcare access than federal politicians. State-level Medicaid expansion, insurance regulations, public options—these happen at state level. Don't ignore local politics.

- **Sustain the pressure.** One phone call doesn't change policy. One town hall doesn't change minds. Sustained, organized pressure over months and years does.

The Treatment Action Campaign in South Africa forced the government to expand access to HIV treatment through sustained pressure over years. They succeeded because they combined moral authority with relentless political mobilization. They didn't give up. They didn't accept incremental symbolic victories. They kept fighting until they won.

That's what winning looks like. Long, hard, sustained organizing that refuses to accept anything less than universal coverage.

The Long Game

Universal healthcare won't happen next year. It might not happen in five years.

But it will happen—if enough people decide to make it happen.

The institutions created to provide universal health coverage are negotiated rather than designed—they're the outcomes of politics and contestation. The UK's NHS, Canada's Medicare, Taiwan's National Health Insurance—all emerged from sustained political struggle against entrenched interests.

In every case, industry opposition was fierce. In every case, politicians claimed it was impossible. In every case, they were wrong—because organized people overcame organized money.

Movement toward universal health coverage is a long-term policy engagement that needs both technical knowledge and political know-how. You now have the technical knowledge from reading this book. The political know-how comes from doing the work.

- Every conversation you have about healthcare is political organizing.
- Every story you share is advocacy.

- Every vote you cast is a statement about what kind of country you want to live in.
- Every call you make to a congressional office is pressure.
- Every town hall you attend is a demonstration of power.
- The system wants you to feel powerless. It wants you to believe that nothing can change, that the forces arrayed against universal healthcare are too powerful, that your individual actions don't matter.

They're lying.

The largest expansion of public health coverage in the United States occurred in the 1960s when the government overcame opposition from groups including the American Medical Association to create Medicare and Medicaid. The AMA predicted disaster. They said Medicare would destroy American healthcare. They were powerful, they were organized, and they spent millions fighting it.

They lost.

They lost because ordinary people organized, voted, and demanded change. They lost because politicians faced more pressure from constituents than from industry lobbying. They lost because the moral case for universal coverage was so overwhelming that opposing it became politically untenable.

It can happen again.

But only if you make it happen.

Start today. Join an organization. Share your story. Register people to vote. Call your representatives. Show up at town halls. Build coalitions. Sustain the pressure.

Don't wait for someone else to fix this. Don't assume that the experts or the politicians or the advocacy organizations will handle it. They won't—not unless you make them.

The path to universal healthcare runs through you. Through your organizing, your advocacy, your votes, your stories, your sustained pressure on politicians who would rather avoid the fight.

Are you willing to fight for it?

Because I promise you this: the healthcare industry is willing to fight to keep it. They're spending hundreds of millions of dollars right now to prevent universal coverage. They're lobbying politicians, funding front groups, spreading propaganda, and doing everything in their power to maintain a system that's killing 68,000 Americans every year while generating record profits.

They're fighting. The question is whether you are too.

The Long View

Like I said, I don't know if we'll achieve universal healthcare in my lifetime, but I know it's coming. Because the current system is unsustainable economically and morally.

Healthcare costs keep rising. Medical bankruptcy keeps destroying families. People keep dying from preventable causes.

At some point, Americans will demand better. Healthcare destabilization creates opportunities for reform. When enough people experience the system's cruelty directly—denied care, medical bankruptcy, loved ones dying from preventable conditions—they become willing to fight for alternatives.

The COVID-19 pandemic demonstrated system failures. Millions lost employer-based insurance during the worst possible time. People avoided care due to cost, worsening outcomes. The pandemic killed an estimated 212,000 additional Americans due to lack of universal coverage—deaths that wouldn't have occurred in countries where healthcare isn't tied to employment or ability to pay.

Brian Thompson's assassination revealed collective rage at system cruelty. That rage will either dissipate—channeled safely into ineffective symbolic actions that change nothing—or it will transform into a sustained political movement demanding universal healthcare.

Which outcome occurs depends on whether we're willing to organize, vote, and fight for it.

The System We Deserve

You know how it works now. You know who it serves. You know what it costs.

American healthcare is sick by design. Every piece of dysfunction serves profit. Every death enriches someone. Every bankruptcy transfers risk from corporations to individuals. Every denial of coverage generates revenue.

We documented the design in this book.

Join organizations demanding universal coverage to change it.

Every major expansion of healthcare coverage in American history—Medicare, Medicaid, the ACA—came from sustained social pressure that made inaction more costly than action. It happened because ordinary people organized, voted, and refused to accept that their suffering was inevitable.

It can happen again.

But only if you make it happen.

Final Thoughts

I'm writing this as a practicing nurse practitioner who has spent over two decades working within this system—and I can't stay silent anymore.

I'm complicit in American healthcare's dysfunction—I work for the machine even as I fight against it. That's the trap we're all caught in: we participate in the system because we have no choice, and our participation sustains it.

We can choose differently. We can demand better. We can build the system that should exist instead of accepting the system we have.

Every other developed nation proves it's possible. The evidence is overwhelming. The path is clear.

The only question is: Are you willing to walk it?

Because I am. I've been on the wrong side long enough. I'm ready to fight for the right side.

Are you?

This book has documented how American healthcare is sick by design. Now it's up to you to help cure it.

The choice is yours. Choose wisely. Choose soon. Because while you're deciding, another 68,000 Americans will die who didn't have to.

And that blood is on all of us—until we choose to stop it.

FINAL THOUGHTS

Now that you've read Sick By Design, there are 3 ways to take action:

1. Get the Introduction to my next book free

Poisoned for Profit exposes how American food is designed to make you sick—using chemicals banned everywhere else.

Free introduction when you subscribe to my Authority Builder newsletter email list.

2. Order ***Sick By Design*** in bulk

Special pricing for healthcare organizations, advocacy groups, labor unions, universities, medical schools, and book clubs.

3. Book me as a speaker

I speak on healthcare system design & policy reform, single-payer advocacy, writing your authority book, and nurse entrepreneurship.

Visit www.studio8twentytwo.com for all three options.

REFERENCES

Chapter 1 Sources

1. Bailey ZD, Krieger N, et al. "Structural Racism and Health Inequities in the USA." Lancet. 2017.

2. Yearby R, Clark B, Figueroa JF. "Structural Racism in Historical and Modern US Health Care Policy." Health Affairs. 2022.

3. Social Security Act 1935 (historical document).

4. Hill-Burton Act 1946 (historical document).

5. Taft-Hartley Act 1947 (historical document).

6. Telesford I, Cotter L, Wager E, Cox C. "How does health spending in the U.S. compare to other countries?" Peterson-KFF Health System Tracker. March 11, 2026. https://www.healthsystemtracker.org/chart-collection/health-spending-u-s-compare-countries/

Chapter 2 Sources

1. Levitt L. "A Backlash Against Health Insurers, Redux." JAMA Health Forum. 2025.

2. Gottlieb JD, Shapiro AH, Dunn A. "The Complexity of Billing and Paying for Physician Care." Health Affairs. 2018.

3. Bundorf MK, Gupta S, Kim C. "Trends in US Health Insurance Coverage During the COVID-19 Pandemic." JAMA Health Forum. 2021.

4. Buchmueller TC, Valletta RG. "Work, Health, and Insurance: A Shifting Landscape." Health Affairs. 2017.

5. Abraham JM, Karaca-Mandic P, Simon K. "How Has the ACA's Medical Loss Ratio Regulation Affected Insurer Behavior?" Medical Care. 2014.

6. Anonymous contributors. Online discussion of healthcare premiums. January 2026. [Personal communications].

Chapter 3 Sources

1. Alpert A, Evans WN, Lieber EMJ, Powell D. "Origins of the Opioid Crisis and Its Enduring Impacts." The Quarterly Journal of Economics. 2022;137(2):1139-1179. doi:10.1093/qje/qjab043.

2. Bowra A, Perez-Brumer A, Forman L, Kohler JC. "Accountability in Global Health Systems: Insights From a Network Analysis of Purdue Pharmaceuticals." Globalization and Health. 2025;21(1):45. doi:10.1186/s12992-025-01140-5.

3. Bowra A, Perez-Brumer A, Forman L, Kohler JC. "Interconnected Influence: Unraveling Purdue Pharmaceutical's Role in the Global Response to the Opioid Crisis." The International Journal on Drug Policy. 2024;133:104604. doi:10.1016/j.drugpo.2024.104604.

4. Wouters OJ. "Lobbying Expenditures and Campaign Contributions by the Pharmaceutical and Health Product Industry in the United States, 1999-2018." JAMA Internal Medicine. 2020;180(5):688-697. doi:10.1001/jamainternmed.2020.0146.

5. Kesselheim AS, Avorn J, Sarpatwari A. "The High Cost of Prescription Drugs in the United States: Origins and Prospects for Reform." JAMA. 2016 Aug 23-30;316(8):858-71. doi:10.1001/jama.2016.11237.

6. Wouters OJ, Denolle C, Wei J, Papanicolas I. "Prices and

Affordability of Essential Medicines in 72 Low-, Middle-, and High-Income Markets." JAMA Health Forum. 2025;6(8): e252043. doi:10.1001/jamahealthforum.2025.2043.

7. Barber MJ, Gotham D, Bygrave H, Cepuch C. "Estimated Sustainable Cost-Based Prices for Diabetes Medicines." JAMA Network Open. 2024;7(3):e243474. doi:10.1001/jamanetworkopen.2024.3474.

8. Galkina Cleary E, Jackson MJ, Zhou EW, Ledley FD. "Comparison of Research Spending on New Drug Approvals by the National Institutes of Health vs the Pharmaceutical Industry, 2010-2019." JAMA Health Forum. 2023;4(4): e230511. doi:10.1001/jamahealthforum.2023.0511.

9. Zhou EW, Jackson MJ, Ledley FD. "Spending on Phased Clinical Development of Approved Drugs by the US National Institutes of Health Compared With Industry." JAMA Health Forum. 2023;4(7):e231921. doi:10.1001/jamahealthforum.2023.1921.

10. Rome BN, Nagar S, Egilman AC, et al. "Simulated Medicare Drug Price Negotiation Under the Inflation Reduction Act of 2022." JAMA Health Forum. 2023;4(1):e225218. doi:10.1001/jamahealthforum.2022.5218.

11. Sullivan SD. "Medicare Drug Price Negotiation in the United States: Implications and Unanswered Questions." Value in Health. 2023;26(3):394-399. doi:10.1016/j.jval.2022.11.015.

12. Reitsma MB, Dusetzina SB, Ballreich JM, Trujillo AJ, Mello MM. "Examining Opportunities to Increase Savings From Medicare Price Negotiations." JAMA Internal Medicine. 2023;183(6):581-588. doi:10.1001/jamainternmed.2023.0763.

13. Vogel M, Kakani P, Chandra A, Conti RM. "Medicare Price Negotiation and Pharmaceutical Innovation Following the

Inflation Reduction Act." Nature Biotechnology. 2024;42(3):406-412. doi:10.1038/s41587-023-02096-w.

Chapter 4 Sources

1. Zhou X, Siegel KR, Ng BP, et al. "Cost-Effectiveness of Diabetes Prevention Interventions Targeting High-Risk Individuals and Whole Populations: A Systematic Review." Diabetes Care. 2020;43(7):1593-1616. doi:10.2337/dci20-0018.

2. Kuo S, Ye W, Wang D, et al. "Cost-Effectiveness of the National Diabetes Prevention Program: A Real-World, 2-Year Prospective Study." Diabetes Care. 2025;48(7):1180-1188. doi:10.2337/dc24-1110.

3. Mohan G, Chattopadhyay SK, Ekwueme DU, et al. "Economics of Multicomponent Interventions to Increase Breast, Cervical, and Colorectal Cancer Screening: A Community Guide Systematic Review." American Journal of Preventive Medicine. 2019;57(4):557-567. doi:10.1016/j.amepre.2019.03.006.

4. Chauhan AS, Prinja S, Srinivasan R, et al. "Cost Effectiveness of Strategies for Cervical Cancer Prevention in India." PloS One. 2020;15(9):e0238291. doi:10.1371/journal.pone.0238291.

5. Jacob V, Chattopadhyay SK, Hopkins DP, et al. "Economics of Community Health Workers for Chronic Disease: Findings From Community Guide Systematic Reviews." American Journal of Preventive Medicine. 2019;56(3):e95-e106. doi:10.1016/j.amepre.2018.10.009.

6. Crandall JP, Dabelea D, Knowler WC, Nathan DM, Temprosa M. "The Diabetes Prevention Program and Its Outcomes Study: NIDDK's Journey Into the Prevention of Type 2

Diabetes and Its Public Health Impact." Diabetes Care. 2025;48(7):1101-1111. doi:10.2337/dc25-0014.

7. Siegel KR, Ali MK, Zhou X, et al. "Cost-Effectiveness of Interventions to Manage Diabetes: Has the Evidence Changed Since 2008?" Diabetes Care. 2020;43(7):1557-1592. doi:10.2337/dci20-0017.

8. Weintraub WS, Daniels SR, Burke LE, et al. "Value of Primordial and Primary Prevention for Cardiovascular Disease: A Policy Statement From the American Heart Association." Circulation. 2011;124(8):967-90. doi:10.1161/CIR.0b013e3182285a81.

9. Hartman M, Martin AB, Benson J, Catlin A, and the National Health Expenditure Accounts Team. "National Health Care Spending In 2023: Growth Accelerated But Remained Below Prepandemic Rates." Health Affairs. 2024;43(12):1798-1808. doi:10.1377/hlthaff.2024.01375.

10. Papanicolas I, Niksch M, Figueroa JF. "Avoidable Mortality Across US States and High-Income Countries." JAMA Internal Medicine. 2025;185(5):583-590. doi:10.1001/jamainternmed.2025.0155.

11. Papanicolas I, Mossialos E, Gundersen A, Woskie L, Jha AK. "Performance of UK National Health Service Compared With Other High Income Countries: Observational Study." BMJ. 2019;367:l6326. doi:10.1136/bmj.l6326.

12. Shaw FE, Asomugha CN, Conway PH, Rein AS. "The Patient Protection and Affordable Care Act: Opportunities for Prevention and Public Health." Lancet. 2014;384(9937):75-82. doi:10.1016/S0140-6736(14)60259-2.

13. Chen SC, Pearson SD. "Policy Framework for Covering Preventive Services Without Cost Sharing: Saving Lives and

Saving Money?" JAMA Internal Medicine. 2016;176(8):1185-9. doi:10.1001/jamainternmed.2016.3052.

14. Song S, White A, Kucik JE. "Use of Selected Recommended Clinical Preventive Services - Behavioral Risk Factor Surveillance System, United States, 2018." MMWR. 2021;70(13):461-466. doi:10.15585/mmwr.mm7013a1.

15. Song S, Kucik JE. "Trends in the Utilization of Recommended Clinical Preventive Services, 2011-2019." American Journal of Preventive Medicine. 2021;61(2):149-157. doi:10.1016/j.amepre.2021.03.010.

16. Hong YR, Jo A, Mainous AG. "Up-to-Date on Preventive Care Services Under Affordable Care Act: A Trend Analysis From MEPS 2007-2014." Medical Care. 2017;55(8):771-780. doi:10.1097/MLR.0000000000000763.

17. Fang H, Frean M, Sylwestrzak G, Ukert B. "Trends in Disenrollment and Reenrollment Within US Commercial Health Insurance Plans, 2006-2018." JAMA Network Open. 2022;5(2): e220320. doi:10.1001/jamanetworkopen.2022.0320.

18. Wolf E, Slosar M, Menashe I. "Assessment of Churn in Coverage Among California's Health Insurance Marketplace Enrollees." JAMA Health Forum. 2022;3(12):e224484. doi:10.1001/jamahealthforum.2022.4484.

19. Einav L, Finkelstein A. "The Risk of Losing Health Insurance in the United States Is Large, and Remained So After the Affordable Care Act." Proceedings of the National Academy of Sciences. 2023;120(18):e2222100120. doi:10.1073/pnas.2222100120.

20. Sommers BD, Gourevitch R, Maylone B, Blendon RJ, Epstein AM. "Insurance Churning Rates for Low-Income Adults Under Health Reform: Lower Than Expected but Still Harmful for

Many." Health Affairs. 2016;35(10):1816-1824. doi:10.1377/hlthaff.2016.0455.

21. Sandhu AT, Heidenreich PA, Borden W, et al. "Value-Based Payment for Clinicians Treating Cardiovascular Disease: A Policy Statement From the American Heart Association." Circulation. 2023;148(6):543-563. doi:10.1161/CIR.0000000000001143.

22. Singh P, Fu N, Dale S, et al. "The Comprehensive Primary Care Plus Model and Health Care Spending, Service Use, and Quality." JAMA. 2024;331(2):132-146. doi:10.1001/jama.2023.24712.

23. Jia L, Meng Q, Scott A, Yuan B, Zhang L. "Payment Methods for Healthcare Providers Working in Outpatient Healthcare Settings." The Cochrane Database of Systematic Reviews. 2021;1:CD011865. doi:10.1002/14651858.CD011865.pub2.

24. Chee TT, Ryan AM, Wasfy JH, Borden WB. "Current State of Value-Based Purchasing Programs." Circulation. 2016;133(22):2197-205. doi:10.1161/CIRCULATIONAHA.115.010268.

25. Dzau VJ, McClellan MB, McGinnis JM, et al. "Vital Directions for Health and Health Care: Priorities From a National Academy of Medicine Initiative." JAMA. 2017;317(14):1461-1470. doi:10.1001/jama.2017.1964.

26. Wang P, Vienneau M, Vogeli C, et al. "Reframing Value-Based Care Management: Beyond Cost Reduction and Toward Patient Centeredness." JAMA Health Forum. 2023;4(6):e231502. doi:10.1001/jamahealthforum.2023.1502.

27. Walensky RP, McCann NC. "Challenges to the Future of a Robust Physician Workforce in the United States." The New England Journal of Medicine. 2025;392(3):286-295.

doi:10.1056/NEJMsr2412784.

28. Hsiang WR, Gross CP, Maroongroge S, Forman HP. "Trends in Compensation for Primary Care and Specialist Physicians After Implementation of the Affordable Care Act." JAMA Network Open. 2020;3(7):e2011981. doi:10.1001/jamanetworkopen.2020.11981.

29. Neprash HT, Golberstein E, Ganguli I, Chernew ME. "Association of Evaluation and Management Payment Policy Changes With Medicare Payment to Physicians by Specialty." JAMA. 2023;329(8):662-669. doi:10.1001/jama.2023.0879.

Chapter 5 Sources

1. Gaffney A, McCormick D. "The Affordable Care Act: Implications for Health-Care Equity." Lancet. 2017;389(10077):1442-1452. doi:10.1016/S0140-6736(17)30786-9.

2. Hampton M, Lenhart O. "Access to Health Care and Mental Health-Evidence From the ACA Preexisting Conditions Provision." Health Economics. 2022;31(5):760-783. doi:10.1002/hec.4473.

3. Shaw FE, Asomugha CN, Conway PH, Rein AS. "The Patient Protection and Affordable Care Act: Opportunities for Prevention and Public Health." Lancet. 2014;384(9937):75-82. doi:10.1016/S0140-6736(14)60259-2.

4. Goodson JD, Shahbazi S, Song Z. "Changes in Coverage Among Non-Elderly Adults With Chronic Diseases Following Affordable Care Act Implementation." PloS One. 2022;17(11):e0278414. doi:10.1371/journal.pone.0278414.

5. Rogers MAM, Kim C, Lee JM, Basu T, Tipirneni R. "Private Insurance Coverage for Diabetes Before and After Enactment

of the Preexisting Condition Mandate of the Affordable Care Act, 2005-2016." American Journal of Public Health. 2019;109(4):562-564. doi:10.2105/AJPH.2018.304933.

6. Huguet N, Angier H, Hoopes MJ, et al. "Prevalence of Pre-Existing Conditions Among Community Health Center Patients Before and After the Affordable Care Act." Journal of the American Board of Family Medicine. 2019 Nov-Dec;32(6):883-889. doi:10.3122/jabfm.2019.06.190087.

7. Zhao J, Zheng Z, Nogueira L, Yabroff KR, Han X. "Preexisting Condition Protections Under the Affordable Care Act: Changes in Insurance Coverage, Premium Contributions, and Out-of-Pocket Spending." Value in Health. 2022;25(8):1360-1370. doi:10.1016/j.jval.2022.01.016.

8. Long SK, Bart L, Karpman M, Shartzer A, Zuckerman S. "Sustained Gains in Coverage, Access, and Affordability Under the ACA: A 2017 Update." Health Affairs. 2017;36(9):1656-1662. doi:10.1377/hlthaff.2017.0798.

9. Glied S, Jackson A. "The Future of the Affordable Care Act and Insurance Coverage." American Journal of Public Health. 2017;107(4):538-540. doi:10.2105/AJPH.2017.303665.

10. Einav L, Finkelstein A. "The Risk of Losing Health Insurance in the United States Is Large, and Remained So After the Affordable Care Act." Proceedings of the National Academy of Sciences. 2023;120(18):e2222100120. doi:10.1073/pnas.2222100120.

Chapter 6 Sources

1. Himmelstein DU, Thorne D, Warren E, Woolhandler S. "Medical Bankruptcy in the United States, 2007: Results of a National Study." The American Journal of Medicine. 2009;122(8):741-6.

2. Dickman SL, Himmelstein DU, Woolhandler S. "Inequality and the Health-Care System in the USA." Lancet. 2017;389(10077):1431-1441.

3. Himmelstein DU, Dickman SL, McCormick D, et al. "Prevalence and Risk Factors for Medical Debt and Subsequent Changes in Social Determinants of Health in the US." JAMA Network Open. 2022;5(9):e2231898.

4. Kluender R, Mahoney N, Wong F, Yin W. "Medical Debt in the US, 2009-2020." JAMA. 2021;326(3):250-256.

5. Paturzo JGR, Hashim F, Dun C, et al. "Trends in Hospital Lawsuits Filed Against Patients for Unpaid Bills Following Published Research About This Activity." JAMA Network Open. 2021;4(8):e2121926.

6. Bernard DM, Selden TM, Fang Z. "The Joint Distribution of High Out-of-Pocket Burdens, Medical Debt, and Financial Barriers to Needed Care." Health Affairs. 2023;42(11):1517-1526.

Chapter 7 Sources

1. Anderson JG, Abrahamson K. "Your Health Care May Kill You: Medical Errors." Studies in Health Technology and Informatics. 2017;234:13-17.

2. Battles J, Azam I, Grady M, Reback K. "Advances in Patient Safety and Medical Liability." Agency for Healthcare Research and Quality. 2017.

3. Kern LM, Reshetnyak E, Colantonio LD, et al. "Association Between Patients' Self-Reported Gaps in Care Coordination and Preventable Adverse Outcomes: A Cross-Sectional Survey." Journal of General Internal Medicine. 2020;35(12):3517-3524.

4. Pinheiro LC, Reshetnyak E, Safford MM, Kern LM. "Racial Disparities in Preventable Adverse Events Attributed to Poor Care Coordination Reported in a National Study of Older US Adults." Medical Care. 2021;59(10):901-906.

5. Doty MM, Tikkanen R, Shah A, Schneider EC. "Primary Care Physicians' Role in Coordinating Medical and Health-Related Social Needs in Eleven Countries." Health Affairs. 2020;39(1):115-123.

6. Kern LM, Safford MM, Slavin MJ, et al. "Patients' and Providers' Views on Causes and Consequences of Healthcare Fragmentation in the Ambulatory Setting: A Qualitative Study." Journal of General Internal Medicine. 2019;34(6):899-907.

7. Penm J, MacKinnon NJ, Strakowski SM, Ying J, Doty MM. "Minding the Gap: Factors Associated With Primary Care Coordination of Adults in 11 Countries." Annals of Family Medicine. 2017;15(2):113-119.

8. Schoen C, Osborn R, Squires D, et al. "New 2011 Survey of Patients With Complex Care Needs in Eleven Countries Finds That Care Is Often Poorly Coordinated." Health Affairs. 2011;30(12):2437-48.

9. Prior A, Vestergaard CH, Vedsted P, et al. "Healthcare Fragmentation, Multimorbidity, Potentially Inappropriate Medication, and Mortality: A Danish Nationwide Cohort Study." BMC Medicine. 2023;21(1):305.

10. Kern LM, Lau JD, Rajan M, et al. "Associations Among Claims-Based Care Fragmentation, Self-Reported Gaps in Care Coordination, and Self-Reported Adverse Events." BMC Health Services Research. 2024;24(1):1045.

Chapter 8 Sources

1. Reuters, Associated Press, Wall Street Journal. "Coverage of Brian Thompson Assassination." December 4-9, 2024.

2. U.S. Senate Permanent Subcommittee on Investigations. "Medicare Advantage Alert: Addressing Vulnerabilities to Achieve High-Quality, Person-Centered Care." October 2023.

3. Levitt LZ, Nwosu C, Ashley RH, Dale SB. "Denial of Prior Authorization Requests and Appeal Outcomes in Medicare Advantage Plans in 2022 and 2023." JAMA Health Forum. 2025;6(2):e245197.

4. UnitedHealth Group. "2023 Annual Report and SEC Filings." Compensation data and financial performance metrics.

5. NORC at the University of Chicago, Emerson College Polling, Economist/YouGov. "National polling on public response to Thompson assassination." December 2024.

6. Kaiser Family Foundation. "Medicare Advantage denial rates and prior authorization data." 2023-2024.

Chapter 9 Sources

1. Glied S. "The State of Health Insurance Coverage and the 2024 Election." JAMA Health Forum. 2024;5(3):e240859.

2. Donohue JM, Cole ES, James CV, et al. "The US Medicaid Program: Coverage, Financing, Reforms, and Implications for Health Equity." JAMA. 2022;328(11):1085-1099.

3. Smith RB, Aboulafia G, Sommers BD. "Who Enrolls in Coverage and Who Remains Uninsured? Medicaid Take-Up Before and After the Affordable Care Act and During

Unwinding." The Milbank Quarterly. 2025;103(2):349-389.

4. Aboulafia G, Gruber J, Sommers BD. "The Past and Future of Medicaid and the Affordable Care Act—Support or Sabotage?" JAMA. 2025;334(2):115-118.

5. Gaffney A, McCormick D. "The Affordable Care Act: Implications for Health-Care Equity." Lancet. 2017;389(10077):1442-1452.

Chapter 10 Sources

1. Mohr DC, Elnahal S, Marks ML, Derickson R, Osatuke K. "Burnout Trends Among US Health Care Workers." JAMA Network Open. 2025;8(4):e255954.

2. Bradford L, Glaser G. "Addressing Physician Burnout and Ensuring High-Quality Care of the Physician Workforce." Obstetrics and Gynecology. 2021;137(1):3-11.

3. Harvey SB, Epstein RM, Glozier N, et al. "Mental Illness and Suicide Among Physicians." Lancet. 2021;398(10303):920-930.

4. Hodkinson A, Zhou A, Johnson J, et al. "Associations of Physician Burnout With Career Engagement and Quality of Patient Care: Systematic Review and Meta-Analysis." BMJ. 2022;378:e070442.

5. Saddawi-Konefka D, Moutier CY, Ehrenfeld JM. "Reducing Barriers to Mental Health Care for Physicians." JAMA. 2025.

6. Makhija H, Davidson JE, Lee KC, et al. "National Incidence of Physician Suicide and Associated Features." JAMA Psychiatry. 2025.

7. Guille C, Sen S. "Burnout, Depression, and Diminished Well-

Being Among Physicians." New England Journal of Medicine. 2024;391(16):1519-1527.

8. West CP, Dyrbye LN, Shanafelt TD. "Physician Burnout: Contributors, Consequences and Solutions." Journal of Internal Medicine. 2018;283(6):516-529.

9. McClafferty HH, Hubbard DK, Foradori D, et al. "Physician Health and Wellness." Pediatrics. 2022;150(5):e2022059665.

Chapter 11 Sources

1. Zhou X, Siegel KR, Ng BP, et al. "Cost-Effectiveness of Diabetes Prevention Interventions Targeting High-Risk Individuals and Whole Populations: A Systematic Review." Diabetes Care. 2020;43(7):1593-1616.

2. Kuo S, Ye W, Wang D, et al. "Cost-Effectiveness of the National Diabetes Prevention Program: A Real-World, 2-Year Prospective Study." Diabetes Care. 2025;48(7):1180-1188.

3. Mohan G, Chattopadhyay SK, Ekwueme DU, et al. "Economics of Multicomponent Interventions to Increase Breast, Cervical, and Colorectal Cancer Screening: A Community Guide Systematic Review." American Journal of Preventive Medicine. 2019;57(4):557-567.

4. Chauhan AS, Prinja S, Srinivasan R, et al. "Cost Effectiveness of Strategies for Cervical Cancer Prevention in India." PloS One. 2020;15(9):e0238291.

5. Jacob V, Chattopadhyay SK, Hopkins DP, et al. "Economics of Community Health Workers for Chronic Disease: Findings From Community Guide Systematic Reviews." American Journal of Preventive Medicine. 2019;56(3):e95-e106.

6. Crandall JP, Dabelea D, Knowler WC, Nathan DM, Temprosa

M. "The Diabetes Prevention Program and Its Outcomes Study: NIDDK's Journey Into the Prevention of Type 2 Diabetes and Its Public Health Impact." Diabetes Care. 2025;48(7):1101-1111.

7. Siegel KR, Ali MK, Zhou X, et al. "Cost-Effectiveness of Interventions to Manage Diabetes: Has the Evidence Changed Since 2008?" Diabetes Care. 2020;43(7):1557-1592.

8. Weintraub WS, Daniels SR, Burke LE, et al. "Value of Primordial and Primary Prevention for Cardiovascular Disease: A Policy Statement From the American Heart Association." Circulation. 2011;124(8):967-90.

9. Telesford I, Cotter L, Wager E, Cox C. "How does health spending in the U.S. compare to other countries?" Peterson-KFF Health System Tracker. March 11, 2026.

10. Papanicolas I, Niksch M, Figueroa JF. "Avoidable Mortality Across US States and High-Income Countries." JAMA Internal Medicine. 2025;185(5):583-590.

11. Papanicolas I, Mossialos E, Gundersen A, Woskie L, Jha AK. "Performance of UK National Health Service Compared With Other High Income Countries: Observational Study." BMJ. 2019;367:l6326.

12. Shaw FE, Asomugha CN, Conway PH, Rein AS. "The Patient Protection and Affordable Care Act: Opportunities for Prevention and Public Health." Lancet. 2014;384(9937):75-82.

13. Chen SC, Pearson SD. "Policy Framework for Covering Preventive Services Without Cost Sharing: Saving Lives and Saving Money?" JAMA Internal Medicine. 2016;176(8):1185-9.

14. Song S, White A, Kucik JE. "Use of Selected Recommended Clinical Preventive Services - Behavioral Risk Factor

Surveillance System, United States, 2018." MMWR. 2021;70(13):461-466.

15. Song S, Kucik JE. "Trends in the Utilization of Recommended Clinical Preventive Services, 2011-2019." American Journal of Preventive Medicine. 2021;61(2):149-157.

16. Hong YR, Jo A, Mainous AG. "Up-to-Date on Preventive Care Services Under Affordable Care Act: A Trend Analysis From MEPS 2007-2014." Medical Care. 2017;55(8):771-780.

17. Fang H, Frean M, Sylwestrzak G, Ukert B. "Trends in Disenrollment and Reenrollment Within US Commercial Health Insurance Plans, 2006-2018." JAMA Network Open. 2022;5(2): e220320.

18. Wolf E, Slosar M, Menashe I. "Assessment of Churn in Coverage Among California's Health Insurance Marketplace Enrollees." JAMA Health Forum. 2022;3(12):e224484.

19. Einav L, Finkelstein A. "The Risk of Losing Health Insurance in the United States Is Large, and Remained So After the Affordable Care Act." Proceedings of the National Academy of Sciences. 2023;120(18):e2222100120.

20. Sommers BD, Gourevitch R, Maylone B, Blendon RJ, Epstein AM. "Insurance Churning Rates for Low-Income Adults Under Health Reform: Lower Than Expected but Still Harmful for Many." Health Affairs. 2016;35(10):1816-1824.

21. Sandhu AT, Heidenreich PA, Borden W, et al. "Value-Based Payment for Clinicians Treating Cardiovascular Disease: A Policy Statement From the American Heart Association." Circulation. 2023;148(6):543-563.

22. Singh P, Fu N, Dale S, et al. "The Comprehensive Primary Care Plus Model and Health Care Spending, Service Use, and

Quality." JAMA. 2024;331(2):132-146.

23. Jia L, Meng Q, Scott A, Yuan B, Zhang L. "Payment Methods for Healthcare Providers Working in Outpatient Healthcare Settings." The Cochrane Database of Systematic Reviews. 2021;1:CD011865.

24. Chee TT, Ryan AM, Wasfy JH, Borden WB. "Current State of Value-Based Purchasing Programs." Circulation. 2016;133(22):2197-205.

25. Dzau VJ, McClellan MB, McGinnis JM, et al. "Vital Directions for Health and Health Care: Priorities From a National Academy of Medicine Initiative." JAMA. 2017;317(14):1461-1470.

26. Wang P, Vienneau M, Vogeli C, et al. "Reframing Value-Based Care Management: Beyond Cost Reduction and Toward Patient Centeredness." JAMA Health Forum. 2023;4(6): e231502.

27. Walensky RP, McCann NC. "Challenges to the Future of a Robust Physician Workforce in the United States." The New England Journal of Medicine. 2025;392(3):286-295.

28. Hsiang WR, Gross CP, Maroongroge S, Forman HP. "Trends in Compensation for Primary Care and Specialist Physicians After Implementation of the Affordable Care Act." JAMA Network Open. 2020;3(7):e2011981.

29. Neprash HT, Golberstein E, Ganguli I, Chernew ME. "Association of Evaluation and Management Payment Policy Changes With Medicare Payment to Physicians by Specialty." JAMA. 2023;329(8):662-669.

Chapter 12 Sources

1. Telesford I, Cotter L, Wager E, Cox C. "How does health spending in the U.S. compare to other countries?" Peterson-KFF Health System Tracker. March 11, 2026.

2. Papanicolas I, Mossialos E, Gundersen A, Woskie L, Jha AK. "Performance of UK National Health Service Compared With Other High Income Countries: Observational Study." BMJ. 2019;367:l6326.

3. Allin S, Marchildon GP. "Canada's Healthcare System." BMJ. 2021;372:m4581.

4. Martin D, Miller AP, Quesnel-Vallée A, et al. "Canada's Universal Healthcare System: Achieving Its Potential." Lancet. 2018;391(10131):1718-1735.

5. Schneider EC, Shah A, Doty MM, et al. "Mirror, Mirror 2021: Reflecting Poorly - Health Care in the U.S. Compared to Other High-Income Countries." Commonwealth Fund. August 2021.

6. Galvani AP, Parpia AS, Foster EM, et al. "Improving the Prognosis of Health Care in the USA." Lancet. 2020;395(10223):524-533.

7. Cai C, Runte J, Ostrer I, et al. "Projected Costs of Single-Payer Healthcare Financing in the United States: A Systematic Review of Economic Analyses." PLoS Medicine. 2020;17(1): e1003013.

8. Pollin R, Heintz J, Arno P, et al. "Economic Analysis of Medicare for All." Political Economy Research Institute, University of Massachusetts-Amherst. November 2018.

9. Himmelstein DU, Woolhandler S. "The Current and Projected Taxpayer Shares of US Health Costs." American Journal of

Public Health. 2016;106(3):449-52.

10. Woolhandler S, Himmelstein DU. "Single-Payer Reform: The Only Way to Fulfill the President's Pledge of More Coverage, Better Benefits, and Lower Costs." Annals of Internal Medicine. 2017;166(8):587-588.

11. Hsiao WC. "Lessons From Taiwan's Universal National Health Insurance: An Interview with William C. Hsiao." Conducted by Ming-Chin Monique Tsai. Interview Quarterly. 2015;6(4): IQ20150407.

12. Cheng TM. "Taiwan's National Health Insurance System: High Value for the Dollar." In: Okma KGH, Crivelli L, editors. Six Countries, Six Reform Models - The Healthcare Reform Experience of Israel, the Netherlands, New Zealand, Singapore, Switzerland and Taiwan. 2009. pp. 171-204.

13. Marchildon GP. "The Crisis of Regionalization." Healthcare Policy. 2015;10(SP):7-9.

14. Mossialos E, Wenzel M, Osborn R, Sarnak D, editors. "2015 International Profiles of Health Care Systems." Commonwealth Fund. January 2016.

15. Cylus J, Figueras J, Normand C. "Will Population Ageing Spell the End of the Welfare State? A Review of Evidence and Policy Options." European Observatory on Health Systems and Policies. 2019.

16. Bevan A. "In Place of Fear." Simon and Schuster. 1952.

17. Gorsky M, Mold A, Martland R. "The NHS and an Ageing Society: Intergenerational Equity or Sustainable Social Contract?" History and Policy. 2016.

18. AMN Healthcare. "New Survey Shows Physician Appointment Wait Times Surge 19% in 2022." AMN Healthcare Press Release. October 24, 2022.

www.ingramcontent.com/pod-product-compliance
Lightning Source LLC
LaVergne TN
LVHW052217200926
848481LV00001B/139
* 9 7 8 1 7 3 6 2 4 8 5 5 3 *